Let's Never Talk About This Again

Let's Never Talk About This Again

A MEMOIR

Sara Faith Alterman

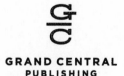

GRAND CENTRAL
PUBLISHING

NEW YORK   BOSTON

Grand Central Publishing
Hachette Book Group
1290 Avenue of the Americas, New York, NY 10104
grandcentralpublishing.com
twitter.com/grandcentralpub

First Edition: June 2020

Grand Central Publishing is a division of Hachette Book Group, Inc. The Grand Central Publishing name and logo is a trademark of Hachette Book Group, Inc.

The publisher is not responsible for websites (or their content) that are not owned by the publisher.

The Hachette Speakers Bureau provides a wide range of authors for speaking events. To find out more, go to www.hachettespeakersbureau.com or call (866) 376-6591.

Library of Congress Cataloging-in-Publication Data has been applied for.

ISBNs: 978-1-5387-4867-1 (hardcover); 978-1-5387-4865-7 (ebook)

Printed in the United States of America

LSC-C

10 9 8 7 6 5 4 3 2 1

For Ira Norman Alterman

Could be worse. Could be raining.

—Mel Brooks

Contents

Foreword

I am pundamentally a word nerd. It comes from my father, or came, I guess. Past tense. He died. But his puns live on posthumorously.

Dad's name is Ira, or was. I don't know if a box of dust can have a name. I guess Ira is as good a name as any for a box of dust.

When I was a kid, our family Volvo was my comedy classroom. We'd pile into that overripe tomato–colored station wagon for quick trips to the ice cream stand in the next town over, or endlessly long trips to the L.L.Bean outlet in Freeport, Maine; Dad would throw me and my brother, Daniel, into a rapid-fire game of wordplay, which had no point but to make each other laugh, or groan. His favorite was a rhyming pun exercise he'd made up to pass the time.

I'll give you an example: One summer our neighbor hired me to walk her dog, Esme, rhymes with "yes, may," which inspired hours of brain twisting.

My father would call back over his shoulder, something like, "What's Esme's favorite condiment?" and you'd screw your face into a constipated prune, trying to contort syllables in your head until you finally came up with the answer: *Esme-onnaise.*

Dad would be so tickled when we figured it out. Well, if. We almost never figured it out. But Dad could go for days. "What would it be called if Esme were a spy? *Esme-ionage!* What's Esme's favorite song? *Esme-rican Pie!* How did Esme's ancestors arrive here? *The Es-Mayflower!*"

This was all happening in Massachusetts. When I was born, we lived in the suburb where the Boston Marathon starts; later, we moved to a historic town that had such a starring role in the American Revolution that the zip code is 01776. And if you think there are no puns to be made about that, it's here that I must Minutemention the varsity-level quip skills we coloneeded to keep up with Dad. I Paul Revere him. I'll stop there.

I ate those word games up with a spoon, so in awe of my dad's quick wit. In many ways I was a junior version of him, or wanted to be. We had the same coarse curly hair, same Silly Putty nose that points to our chin when we smile. Smiled. We were both wild for Chuck Berry records and Mel Brooks movies, and I loved Dad so blindly that it took me ten years to realize he'd shaped my tastes on purpose.

It took me another ten years to realize that our favorite Mel Brooks movie, *Young Frankenstein*, has a sex scene at the end. I'd always assumed it ended, kind of abruptly, on Madeline Kahn brushing her hair at a vanity table while singing "The Battle Hymn of the Republic," which is when my father would spring from our scratchy brown couch to jab the stop button on the VCR.

The first time I watched *Young Frankenstein* as a young adult—in my French vanilla concrete dorm room, freshman year of college—I learned that it does not end after Madeline Kahn brushes her hair while singing, "Mine eyes have seen the glory of the coming of the Lord." It ends after Madeline Kahn squirms beneath Peter Boyle while singing, "Oh, sweet mystery of life, at last I've found you."

I didn't ask Dad why he'd never let me watch the full ending of *Young Frankenstein*, because I didn't have to. This was a man who was allergic to difficult conversation and made us say "bottom" instead of "butt." A man who grounded me for two weeks when he caught me with a cup of coffee before I turned sixteen, the age he'd sanctioned as coffee-ready. A man who did whatever he could to protect his kids from prematurely becoming adults.

He was also a man who picked me up from every ballet class with a carton of chocolate milk and a package of peanut butter crackers, who taught me to drive his car in the snow, and, years later, drove thirty miles to dig mine out in a blizzard.

And he was a man who eventually lost his wonderful words, driving privileges, and social graces to Alzheimer's disease. No longer burdened by the need to filter the world for the benefit of his children, Dad finally spoke openly and honestly about something he'd kept hidden from us for our entire lives; an open secret that I didn't have the stomach, or balls, to talk about, until conversations with my father had an expiration date.

More on all of this later.

For now, all you need to know is that I loved my dad so much. Love. Present tense.

Part I
Before

Chapter 1

THE DUCK ROOM

The most important room in my childhood home was covered in ducks; a first-floor den that we called the Duck Room.

I worked in branding for a while, coming up with names for products and start-ups and buildings, and there was one guy at my company who would get so frustrated during brainstorming sessions that he would finally yell, "Call it what it is! Why are we fucking around with this, guys? We should just call it what it is!" Of course, if we always called things what they were, the world would be full of Overhyped Pink Wines, and I *Can* Believe It's Not Butters, and Sneakers for Elves at Raves.

But in this case, the "Duck Room" captures it perfectly. The room had wallpaper with a mallard pattern that was as tasteful a mallard pattern as a mallard pattern could be. I remember the paper as red, but my mom insists it was brown. Armchairs were upholstered with another tasteful duck pattern that Mom and I both agree was yellow. Our duck-shaped phone had a curly black cord extruding uncomfortably from her fine-feathered bottom. It was all pretty classy for the mid-1980s.

The Duck Room was important because it was the nerve center

of our house: part media library, part family archives, where we kept all of our games, records, VHS tapes, photo albums, and books. Our TV was in there, and our VCR, and a convertible "flip chair" that was just wide enough for me and Daniel to cuddle up on together when our family settled in to watch a show or movie. Mom usually took the couch, and Dad liked the armchair closest to the TV, just in case a racy scene came on and he had to spring into action, changing the channel or jabbing at the fast-forward button on the VCR. The Duck Room was my favorite place in the house.

It was also where my image of my dad changed forever. Alterman, forever altered, man.

I'll show myself out.

The room had two floor-to-ceiling built-in bookcases that flanked a sliding glass door leading out to our deck, where our three cats that I always forget about liked to sleep in the sun. I always forget about them because they were outdoor cats, and belonged to the woods, and knew that they were better than us. Their names were China, Tasha, and Sunday, and sometimes my dad would catch a glimpse of one of them and start singing "Memory," the only song he could stand from the Broadway musical *Cats*.

The built-ins had storage cabinets at the base, and those jutted out far enough that there was room for me or Daniel to stand on top of them when we wanted something from a shelf. I could reach every shelf except the top one. It was an easy climb, and from there we could explore a hodgepodge of cookbooks, novels, storybooks, and random artifacts from our parents' lives before they were our parents: like newspaper clippings, their high school yearbooks, an invitation from First Lady Rosalynn Carter that requested the pleasure of my father's company at some dinner for employees of senior citizen–related publications, which, at one point in his life, he was.

I loved the yearbooks, loved seeing the kinds of kids my parents had been. My teenage mom looked like a young Penelope Cruz with a Jackie Kennedy hairdo. There are photos of her throughout, some where she'd posed with her choirs and clubs, and one candid from a fancy-looking dance, where she looks stunning but uncomfortable. Mom sang soprano with the madrigal singers, and even went to All-State one year. Above her class portrait it reads *Chords that vibrate sweetest pleasure.*

Dad's yearbook was called *The Pennridge High School Pennant.* He's wearing thick Buddy Holly glasses in his class portrait, and above it reads *Gift of self-expression... quotable... way out humor... strong convictions... irrepressible.*

Even on my tiptoes on top of the cabinet, I couldn't reach higher than the second-highest shelf, but that was fine. I kept most of my own books in my bedroom, and never really *needed* anything from the Duck Room, except my own cookbooks, and a rainbow-colored set of kids' encyclopedias called *The Childcraft How and Why Library.* It was a collection of a dozen or so volumes like *Mathemagic*, which combined arithmetic lessons with puzzles, games, and stories, including the tale of a little boy named Milo, who travels to a magical world and meets a friendly human-like shape with twelve faces: the Dodecahedron. Each face showed a different expression, and when his mood changed, they would shuffle around. I loved this little creature, and the idea that you could have ever-changing moods all over your body, like a blush in your armpit, or a frown on your knee. I read and reread the Dodecahedron's story for years before I found out that it was an excerpt from the fantasy novel *The Phantom Tollbooth.*

Instead of being excited that there was so much more to Milo's story, I was gutted! What do you *mean*, my favorite story was just *one small part* of another story? This whole time I could have been reading about *bigger* adventures, with *more* wonderful creatures? I felt cheated, like I'd missed out on years of opportunities to develop a deeper and more complete connection with something I loved. It made me wonder what else I was missing out on.

I'd already suspected that there was a wide, wild world beyond the Duck Room. Even though my own shelves were stocked with G-rated material, I had a few friends who were allowed to see PG-rated movies, *without* their parents present for guidance. That blew my mind. And made me jealous.

Out of curiosity, or maybe defiance, or maybe even in an act of quiet mutiny, I began to snoop through my parents' shelves and drawers when they weren't paying attention, just to see if, like *Mathemagic*, they were holding anything back from me, too.

I didn't find anything interesting, not on purpose. One humdrum Saturday, while my parents were at the grocery store, I scaled the Duck Room bookcase to grab my copy of *The Sesame Street Cookbook*, so Mom and I could make Snuffle Loaf in a Spaghetti Nest together for dinner.

While I was up there, I noticed that I was finally tall enough to reach the top shelf. A whole new trove of goodies to explore.

First I found a fancy wooden book that wasn't a book at all, but a blue-velvet-lined case containing a few intricately carved tobacco pipes. Next, a small red book with pages that crackled with age. My mom's teenage diary. I did a quick flip through; she mostly wrote about some guy who she wanted to take her skiing. Then, they went skiing.

Way in the corner of the shelf, I found a stash of tall, thin paperbacks packed tightly together—and, behind them, there were a few more, hidden from plain sight. I crammed my fingers between two spines so I could wiggle one of the books out of the sardined pack.

There was an orange cartoon cat—sort of a poor man's Garfield—on the cover. She was scraggly and orange, with heavy pink eyelids and softly floppy whiskers that reminded me of overcooked spaghetti. The cat sat, human-style, leaning on her elbows in front of a checkerboard, looking about as interested in *it* as our snooty cats were in *us*. It was called *Games You Can Play with Your Pussy*.

A book about games! I loved games! Why hadn't I seen it before? Why was it shoved out of reach?

I cracked *Games You Can Play with Your Pussy* open and found that it was a chapter book, divided into sections like "How to Clean Your Pussy," "How to Feed Your Pussy," and "Nursing a Sick Pussy." That one begins: *Nothing looks quite so sad as a sick pussy. The spunk, the vitality, the old get-up-and-go have all got up and gone.*

But...there weren't any games in this game book. And the how-to chapters didn't contain any actual grooming or feeding information. I knew that *my* cats disdainfully licked themselves clean and ate bowls of colorful, crunchy bits shaped like tiny drumsticks and three-leaf clovers with no stems.

I stuck my fingers back into the pack and wiggled a few more books out. There was *So You've Got a Fat Pussy!*, with a cartoon cover cat that looked like it had eaten the first one. *How to Pick Up Men* featured a blond woman in a slinky dress. A man in a green suit sat in her lap—a *man* sitting in a *lady's* lap?! Hilarious! And two other men in the background, looking askance.

It took a little effort to wiggle out the hidden books, but I finally managed to get a few loose. They had names like *The Official Italian Sex Manual*, *Sex Manual for People over 30*, and *The*

Jewish Sex Manual. And there was one with a very eye-catching cover, called *Bridget's Sexual Fantasies.*

I'd never heard the word "sexual" before, but I did love the Disney movie *Fantasia.*

On the cover of *Bridget's Sexual Fantasies* was a photograph of a large, topless woman with ripe apple cheeks and juicy watermelon breasts, holding a braided rope and some kind of lacy belt. She looked up at something, or someone, beyond the camera. She looked happy.

Something below my stomach gave a little *ping!* Cautiously, I opened the book. It was full of photos of the same large woman, the "Bridget" of the title, spilling out of different skimpy costumes, posing with different smiling men. As I flipped through the pages, I found many more words I didn't recognize. "Bondage." "Voyeurism." "Orgy." One unfamiliar term, "Oral Sex," was at the top of a story about lollipops. I started to read it, but then I heard the garage door rumble, announcing my parents' return, so I hurried to shove the books back into their place on the top shelf. My father got mad whenever we messed with his stuff, and based on how the books were shelved, I got the feeling that I wasn't supposed to be looking at them.

As I hurried to put everything back into what I hoped was the same order I'd found it in, some familiar words caught my eye. More precisely, a familiar name.

The first page of *Games You Can Play with Your Pussy* said, "by Ira Alterman."

That couldn't be right.

Ira Alterman. That's my father's name.

I knew I was seconds away from being caught red-handed, but I couldn't resist checking the title pages of the other books: *So You've Got a Fat Pussy!*, by Ira Alterman. *How to Pick Up*

Men, by Ira Alterman. *Bridget's Sexual Fantasies*, as told to Ira Alterman.

The *ping!* below my stomach turned into a brick. *What. The. H-e-double hockey sticks?*

There was barely time to process this fresh and confusing information before I heard a noise in the hallway and realized that—*oh no!*—someone was coming. I jammed those books back into place as fast as I could, jumped down from the cabinet, and landed with an ungraceful *THUD* just as Dad appeared in the doorway.

"What are you doing?" he asked.

For a second I thought about asking Dad about these confusing books, but I didn't want to get in trouble for touching his things. For now, I'd pretend I hadn't seen them.

"Just getting my cookbook," I said, and quickly grabbed *The Sesame Street Cookbook* from its familiar place on the shelf. "And, um, looking at your yearbook."

"Ha! That old thing," Dad said. "Have I ever told you about the time I had to play the piano in a jazz band at a talent show? It was last-minute. I didn't even play the piano, but I had to figure it out as I went. They call that '*out-on-a-limb*-provisation.'"

And then we took *The Sesame Street Cookbook* into the kitchen, and Mom helped me shape a lump of ground meat into the suggestion of a Snuffleupagus. The whole time, questions about the books tumbled around in my head, and I wasn't sure how to ask them, or even if I should.

So, I didn't. I kept everything I knew and wondered about these strange books to myself. For the next twenty-five years.

Chapter 2

HEAR YE, HEAR YE

Dad's name didn't belong in those books. They didn't even belong in our bookshelves.

My parents, Ira and Carolyn, were straitlaced squares who wouldn't have let me or Daniel anywhere near a book with a naked lady in it. They were sticklers for rules—and our house had a *lot* of rules. No listening to music that hadn't been pre-vetted, no PG-13 movies until we actually turned thirteen. We couldn't say "butt" or "fart," or watch kissing scenes, or eat sugary cereal unless we were on vacation. They wanted to protect us from anything that would rot our brains, teeth, or innocence, and their expectations for us were very clear: Keep it squeaky clean. We were allowed a little leeway on holidays. My brother always asked for two swears as his birthday present, and, permission granted, he'd stand at the top of the stairs and gleefully bellow: "HELL! DAMN!" I don't think he dared go any bluer. Dad would wince and look down at the floor, shaking his head at the pleasure his little boy took in those big words.

Overall, my parents created a whimsical, wholesome world for our family, and we had a lot of fun together. Dad lived for grand gestures, loved to totally blow our minds with over-the-top birthday cakes and elaborate Christmas mornings. "Santa" always wrote clever clues on our gift tags, and we'd have to guess at what was beneath the wrapping paper before we tore in. "It's time for a present" might be the tag on a cute alarm clock, or "Doll in the family" on a Cabbage Patch Kid.

My dad even gave me a purity ring, with literal fanfare. To be (fan)fair, he didn't have God in mind when he bought the jewelry that was supposed to symbolize chastity. He didn't even believe in God.

In the second grade I was desperate for a ring just like the one my best friend Allie wore on her left hand. The delicate gold band seemed so much more sophisticated than my own stick-on earrings, or the bulbous silver heart necklace I'd put a dent in with my back teeth.

Allie said she wore the ring because she'd made a promise to God to stay pure. I didn't understand what that meant, and I'm not sure she did either. What do little girls know about purity, besides the shameless, shameful pressures that their parents or religions heap upon them? I begged my parents for a thin gold ring so that I, too, could make a purity promise to God.

"The only promise you're making to God," said my father, an atheist Jew, "is that if he comes anywhere near you, he's getting a knuckle sandwich."

I put the ring out of my mind. But Dad must have liked the symbolism of it.

Every fall my parents took us to King Richard's Faire, a seasonal medieval fantasy in a southeastern Massachusetts forest, featuring an artisan marketplace, blacksmith demonstrations, wandering minstrels, juggling fools, swaggering knights, pony rides, ax throwing competitions, a zoo for some reason, and food stalls that offered juicy turkey legs served by juicier maidens. I loved those turkey legs. Daniel loved those maidens.

That final "e" in "faire" is an important distinction. There are *fairs*, like festivals of fried food, agricultural competitions, and barfy Tilt-A-Whirls; and then there are *faires*, carnivals of jousting and mead flagons and jesters going to night school to become radiology technicians. Disneyland for people who love chain mail and being referred to as *m'lady*.

It was—no, *'twas* here one crisp and sunny October afternoon that I was gallivanting about in a felt princess hat that looked like an upside-down ice cream cone with a trailing tail of tulle, while Daniel swung a plastic sword around at an imaginary dragon, when—behold!—I heard a ballyhoo of trumpets behind me.

"Good Lady Sara!" boomed a double bass voice, and I spun around to find a noble and bearded silver fox in a brocaded tunic, speaking directly to…me. It was the king. *The* king. King Richard. His wife, Queen Can't Remember Her Name, stood by his side, a total babe in a tall gold tiara.

"Your…Majesty," I said, in awe of his local celebrity. A murmuring crowd began to gather. They may have wondered if this was part of the show, if this gobsmacked little girl would be revealed to be a secret warrior witch princess.

"Lady Sara," the king said, "'tis my royal pleasure to present thee with a treasure from the court. May thou cherish it always."

Then the trumpets played again and a man with a little red pillow appeared, and on that pillow perched my birthday present: a thin and delicate gold ring.

I was over the moon about this surprise, giving the king a thousand hugs. My parents let him take the credit, maybe because they'd already said no to the ring and didn't want to look weak. I put it on the third finger of my left hand and took any opportunity to wave my hand around to show it off, like a newly engaged woman.

Allie was thrilled about my new jewelry, too, because it meant we were twins! Schoolgirls love to be twins! We held our hands next to each other to compare rings, hers perfectly round, mine a series of angles, like a stop sign with no middle. She was also thrilled that I'd made a twinsie promise to God, and I didn't tell her the truth, that a king gave me jewelry with no sanctimonious strings attached.

I didn't even know what I was supposed to be promising anyway. Virginity? Abstinence? I didn't know what those things were. A promise to avoid the topic of sex altogether? In the second grade, I didn't know what that was either. Any questions I might have had about those forbidden movies and kissing scenes were brushed off or ignored. Sometimes it felt like the whole world was off-limits.

It's not like Daniel and I were locked in a windowless basement with a pile of *Highlights* magazines and only each other for company. It's more that our parents were ferocious watchdogs of culture. So, while my Esprit-clad friends were singing Madonna songs into their hairbrushes or taping Michael J. Fox posters to their bedroom walls, I was belting Judy Collins classics in the bubble bath, and writing fan letters to Ben Vereen, the iconic Broadway actor who played the singing, dancing civil servant snow leopard Mayor Ben on *Zoobilee Zoo*.

I didn't know it was weird for an elementary school '80s kid to have a baby boomer's taste in music. I just liked what I liked, which was what my parents liked. We had a record player in the living room, along with a massive album collection. Mom taught me about show tunes and operas and musicals, like *The Three-penny Opera, Show Boat, Camelot.* Dad liked any genre, as long as it had a beat, but he was especially moved by Dave Brubeck, Dizzy Gillespie, Fats Waller, Fats Domino, and Chuck Berry. His favorite Chuck Berry song was "Johnny B. Goode," and Daniel and I loved it too. We'd bop around the living room until it was done, then scurry to drag the needle back to the opening notes over and over again, making my father anxious that we'd scratch the record or wear it out.

Around the same time that Dad gave me the gold ring—about a year before I found the books—my music teacher at school had our class go around in a circle and name our favorite songs. Other kids listed stuff I'd never heard of, by bands like Bon Jovi and U2 and the Bangles.

When it was my turn, I blurted, "'Johnny B. Goode'!" to an audience of confused crickets. Finally, Allie said: "Oh, from *Back to the Future!*" and then the room got rowdy, and then *I* was confused.

"From *what?*" I asked.

"*Back to the Future*," said one of the three kids named Adam. "The *movie?*"

"I got the tape for my birthday," said another Adam. "I've probably watched it fifty times. You've *never* seen it?"

With kids it's one false move and you're the dummy of the day, so I pretended to know what everyone was talking about. "Oh...yeah," I said, trying to sound annoyed with his stupidity. "A-*doy*. A-doy *hickey*."

That was enough to convince Allie and all three Adams that I also absolutely knew about and had definitely seen *Back to the Future*. I nodded along as my friends chattered about how cool it was when Marty McFly totally smoked the guitar at an enchanted dance under the sea.

"Wicked cool!" I added, doubling down on my smoke screen and my Massachusetts-ness. "Wicked cool."

Of course, I'd never seen *Back to the Future*. The Duck Room was stocked with Disney cartoons like *The Sword in the Stone*, *Swiss Family Robinson*, and *Robin Hood*, starring a foxy fox that I had a crush on, and live-action stuff like *Shelley Duvall's Faerie Tale Theatre* and *The Apple Dumpling Gang*.

"So, um," I asked, so totally super casually that I accidentally dribbled spit into my own long hair, "what other stuff are you guys into right now?"

Electrified, my little friends chattered about movies and music and people I'd never heard of. I tried to take mental notes. The easiest name for me to remember was Jon Bon Jovi, because of the way it rhymed. It reminded me of something I'd come up with as part of a road-trip word game.

When my father got home that night I asked him, "Can I see *Back to the Future*?"

"No way, José," he said.

"But 'Johnny B. Goode' is in it!" I protested. "Did you know Chuck Berry didn't actually write that song? He got the idea from Marty McFly when they were at a party underwater."

"Where did you hear that?" he asked.

"My friends. Everyone's seen it but me."

My father shook his head. "Listen," he said. "Those kids are knuckleheads. Their parents are letting them watch garbage. Chuck Berry wrote that song, not some floppy-haired pipsqueak in a tweed jacket."

I hung my head in disappointment, but then—

"Wait," I said. "How do you know what Marty McFly looked like? Have *you* seen *Back to the Future*?!"

"No," he said. I let it go, but *man*, was that unfair. How was I going to keep up at school if I couldn't do the same stuff as my friends? Ugh. School is like keeping up with the junior Joneses, you know? And I already felt like I was one bulky sweat suit away from being a total outcast.

Besides curating our music and movies, my parents were a two-person approval committee for clothes and shoes. We mostly shopped at outlet malls or department stores like Bradlees and Caldor. I loved the department stores because I could slip away from my parents as they flipped through racks of turtlenecks and piles of bulky jeans that my mom called "dungarees," and go look longingly at things I wasn't allowed to buy, like press-on nails and off-the-shoulder T-shirts.

The next time my parents took us shopping, I slipped into the music section to look for the bands my friends gushed about. I pulled Bon Jovi's *Slippery When Wet* from a bin and brought it to my mom. Maybe, oh-so-hopefully, all I'd need to do to experience music outside the realm of my parents' taste was ask.

"Can I get this?" I asked optimistically.

Mom flipped the tape over to read the back cover. "Oh no, I don't *think* so," she said disdainfully. "You are *not* getting something that has a song called 'Social *Disease.*'"

I didn't know what a social disease was, but Mom seemed so disgusted that I didn't want to push it. Maybe it was, like, really bad, like the Black Spot in Robert Louis Stevenson's *Treasure Island*. I'd never actually read it, but we had it on tape, and I always imagined the Black Spot as an open sore that you'd slip into someone's hand, like a coin, or an extra cookie.

"But Mom!" I pleaded. "Everyone at school has it!"

"I find *that* hard to believe," she said.

"This is so *unfair!*" I whined, and just then my dad walked up. "What's so unfair?" he asked.

Mom gestured to me with the tape. "She wants me to *buy* her a *tape* with a song called '*Social Disease.*'"

"That garbage? I don't *think* so," Dad said, unknowingly echoing my mother. I wondered if, after a decade of marriage and raising kids together, their brains had simply melded.

I didn't get to find out what a social disease was, because my father snatched that tape out of my hands and tossed it right on the ground. It skidded beneath a table piled with geometric sweaters, and I didn't dare pick it up.

Chapter 3

UCK, FEH.

I don't like to talk about it much, but my father had a fiery temper. You could tell when he was about to blow because his nostrils would flare like a fighting bull's, and then *BAM!* He'd throw something across the room, or say something incredibly mean. It often happened when he was stressed out, or if Daniel and I messed with his stuff, or asked about something that made Dad uncomfortable.

Dad's day job was to help people navigate difficult conversations. He worked for a company that produced executive education programs, and he led the program development and marketing teams, organizing and promoting weeklong conferences led by professors from elite universities, who would teach subjects like negotiation tactics and conflict resolution. I think that's right. To be honest, he was pretty vague about it.

The great irony of my father making his living from helping people to deal with difficult conversations was that *he* couldn't. Dad was practically allergic to awkwardness, and whenever he felt squeamish he'd screw up his face and say, "Uck, feh," like he'd just found something gross on the bottom of his shoe. Dad would *uck, feh* at gooey pop music on the radio, at people kissing in the mall, at those forbidden love scenes on TV. He'd change the station as fast as he could. There were no remote controls then, or at least we didn't own any remote-controlled things, so he'd have to make a great, weird leap from wherever he was sitting. Once, he couldn't get the VCR to cooperate, so he pulled the plug out of the wall.

I didn't understand, and still don't understand, why something as benign as a kissing scene made my father uncomfortable. He was so weird about it, and *so* committed to being weird about it, that I grew to find those scenes uncomfortable too. But the books with Dad's name in them seemed to have their fair share of kissing stuff, plus some body-part sucking stuff, and a lot of crying out. Maybe body-part sucking is painful.

I was afraid to bring it up, because whenever my father felt backed into a corner by a topic that made him uncomfortable, or by a situation that made him feel like he'd lost control, he'd go bonkers. I think it was his way of showing the family who was in charge.

One night Dad brought home a new home stereo, with a record player and built-in cassette deck. As he unpacked it, he announced that he'd be transferring all of his albums over to tapes. He started with *Chuck Berry's Golden Hits*. The sleeve featured an exuberant blond lady, mid-shimmy in a low-cut sequined dress, posing provocatively beneath a colorful list of the tracks. Sometimes when I danced to "Roll Over Beethoven," I shook my bottom extra hard and pretended to be her.

Dad stuck a cassette into the deck, started the album, hit the record button, and headed into the kitchen to grab his favorite end-of-the-workweek drink; neon-green Midori on the rocks. Daniel and I did our usual bopping around to "Johnny B. Goode." When it was over I excitedly dragged the needle back to the beginning. Immediately, Dad ran in from the kitchen and lost his mind.

"You ruined the recording!" he yelled. "Now I have to start the whole thing over again!" And he hurled the album cover across the room. The exuberant blond lady hit our brick fireplace face-first, and I took off running for the emotional safety of my bedroom.

About an hour later, Dad rapped gently on my door. He came in, apologized for losing his temper, and tossed the transferred Chuck Berry cassette onto my bed.

"That's for you," he said. "A little pressie, to say I'm sorry."

He always did that in the aftermath of an explosion: came in to apologize—sotto voce and contrite—and to give me a present, or a cookie, or a bowl of ice cream. And then we'd hug, and pretend the blowup never happened.

It was deeply confusing to grow up with a father who could snap in an instant, especially because I wanted to be his shadow, his little double. I felt his affection, but I never felt fully comfortable with his unpredictable moods. Maybe it would have been easier for me to reconcile these clashing faces of Dad if I'd thought of them in terms of my beloved Dodecahedron, who had a front-facing sweet face and other, secret faces that nobody else could see unless he spun around. But I was a kid and didn't think like that. Instead, I just tried to avoid making my father mad.

These are all reasons why I never brought up those dirty books with the busty women, and Dad's name on the title pages. I knew it would be the ultimate difficult conversation, that he'd realize he wasn't controlling the narrative with his kids anymore. I was afraid he'd throw the books against the wall. Or, worse, take them away.

Although I never talked about *Bridget's Sexual Fantasies*, or *Games You Can Play with Your Pussy*, or *How to Pick Up Men*, I sure did read them a lot.

I can't explain why I was drawn to these books when I was still so young. Well, except for the ones about cats. I didn't realize that there were jokes to them that I wasn't getting. I took every line about pussy caretaking at face value and wanted to try out some of these "tips" on our own cats, but I couldn't figure out *how*, exactly. It was hard to interpret the workout regimens in the chapter called "Exercising Your Pussy," which begins:

> They took a poll once to find out what people hate the most. And do you know what finished right behind taxes and the metric system? Flabby pussies.
>
> Yes, all of us agree there is nothing much more useless than a flabby pussy. Pussies ought to be sleek and firm and taut and sinuous. They ought to be. Sometimes they are not. You can fix that, though, by exercising your pussy.

That made sense. We had three flabby pussies at my house. Well, Sunday wasn't too bad, but China and Tasha were both pretty plump. Their favorite thing to do was to lie around in the sun. The book recommended that I run my pussy ragged, but I wasn't sure how to do that. Could you put a cat on a leash? How do you get a leash? I didn't want to ask Mom or Dad to drive me to the pet store, because then I'd have to admit that I knew about the books. The chapter called "Talking with Your Pussy" seemed more doable, but then, under the heading "How to Go About It," it says:

You may not think this is going to work, but all I can say is try it.

Roll a cucumber in yeast, then stroke it gently but firmly until it gets warm and moist and begins to rise. Roll the turgid tuber with cat nip, then smear on a greasy unguent and pack the practically pulsating pickle in a pint of peach preserves. Wave the warm concoction under your pussy's nose so that it understands what's at stake here, then gently suggest to the quivering creature that unless it makes with a few choice sentences, you're going to stick it in her ear.

Yikes. That seemed like a lot.

"Pack the practically pulsating pickle in a pint of peach pre-serves." It reminded me of a road-trip word game that Dad liked to lead, where we'd have to answer a question with a full sentence, in which all of the words began with the same letter.

"Altermans adore alliteration!" he'd hoot, and then pose some nonsense question that would strike me silent for minutes at a time, as I was so, so careful to choose the right words for my answer and follow the rules of the game.

The Bridget books, well. Even an innocent goober like me understood that they were naughty. Bridget wasn't the first naked woman I'd seen. I had a friend, a precocious equestrian named Missy, who showed me an issue of *Playboy* that she'd found in her father's bureau. We spent an entire sleepover flipping through it and comparing our barely there breasts with page after page of sun-caressed sirens blessed with juicy globes and candy kisses for nipples.

But Bridget was *ample*, and she seemed unapologetic. I couldn't stop staring at her. I would sneak little snippets of her stories whenever I could. She just looked so dang *happy*. I wanted to understand why. As far as I could tell, it was largely because she had such fun times with her pilot, doctor, and businessman friends.

A year after discovering the books, I still couldn't make sense of them. *Bridget's Sexual Fantasies* said "As told to Ira Alterman," but who *was* she, and why did she need someone to write down her stories? Maybe she couldn't type? That couldn't be right. There's a whole chapter in *Bridget's Sexual Fantasies* about her career as a secretary.

One day during recess, a girl named Danielle pulled a piece of grass out of my hair and told me that I looked like I had just gone for a roll in the hay.

"What hay? It's just grass," I said, and she laughed.

"Oh my god," she said. "You don't know what 'roll in the hay' means?"

"Yes I do," I said, and told her about a scene in *Young Franken-stein* where an adorable Teri Garr asks Gene Wilder if he'd like to go for a roll in the hay, and then she rolls around in some hay.

But Danielle rolled her eyes. "It's not actually about *rolling around* in *hay*," she said, so *totally over* what an *idiot baby* she had to deal with. "It's, you know," she whispered knowingly, "S...E...X?"

I spelled it in my head. "Oh," I said. "I know that."

She didn't believe me, and why should she have? Of course, I didn't know that. I still didn't really know what S...E...X was.

By middle school my family had moved to a new house in a new town, a historic but progressive suburb of Boston where Revolutionary War soldiers are buried in a hillside cemetery, and the town's oldest building dates to 1730. I thought maybe without a Duck Room, I wouldn't have access to Dad's books anymore. But no—our new house had built-in bookshelves, too, and my parents put everything away in the exact same places they'd been in the old house. *Games You Can Play, How to Pick Up Men, Bridget's Sexual Fantasies*—they were all just as poorly hidden and easily accessible as they'd been in the Duck Room, which was a huge relief.

Also a huge relief? The year my middle school class started sex education, and I could finally make sense of the pussy games, and the fantasies, and the S...E... X.

Chapter 4

SARA OF THE 01776

Kids needed a signed permission slip from their parents in order to participate in sex ed. Anyone whose parents declined to sign, my teacher said, would spend the class period in the library instead.

When I showed the slip to Mom, she immediately deflected and redirected. "Better ask your father when he gets home," she said, and my stomach felt thick. Usually whenever Mom sent me to ask Dad about something, it was because she was nervous about saying yes.

If by now you're thinking that my dad sounds like a bully, you're kind of right. I mean, yes. Clearly, his reaction to stress, especially stress caused by his children, was insanely inappropriate. Now I'm far enough removed that I can sympathize with the kind of pressure he must have felt in trying to keep a secret from us. Maybe that's too generous and forgiving.

When Dad pulled into the driveway that evening, I brought the slip outside. He rolled down his window to say hello, and before he had a chance to get out of the car, I shoved the form in his face.

I just wanted to get it over with. I knew how uncomfortable

he'd be with this form, that he'd *uck, feh* the moment he saw the word "sex" on the page. Maybe even refuse to sign it. I didn't know how many kids at school would be allowed to take the class, but I didn't want to be on the outside looking in *again*, for McFly's sake. I didn't want to add "sex" to the list of things my friends all seemed to know about, while, for me, it remained a mystery.

When I showed the slip to Dad, I tried to joke about it. "This is so *lame*, Dad," I said, rolling my eyes. "They want us to learn about how *little bundles of joy* came to *be*."

I'd seen in one of my mother's supermarket magazines that "little bundle of joy" meant a baby, plus one of my friends told me that her mom and dad "did sexies" to make her baby sister. S…E…X led to little bundles of joy. Duh. Sex ed would be an easy A.

Dad signed that permission slip through his open car window without a single word—without even looking me in the eye.

"How they came to *be*, Dad," I said, trying to keep the joke going. Well, it wasn't really going. But, oops, then *Dad* was going. He put the car in reverse, backed right on out of the driveway, and didn't come back until after dinner.

I'd been right to be worried about feeling left out. Except for one girl whose parents forbade her from it for religious reasons, the whole class was present for sex ed. The teacher didn't divide us by gender, didn't apologize, and didn't bat an eye at our collective humiliation. It was all very clinical. We learned about pubic hair and periods, the vas deferens and sperm, and ejaculation and fertilization. There was lots of reproductive system talk: Here's a penis, here's a vagina; stop laughing at the word "vagina"; every month one ovary releases a—*stop* laughing at the word "vagina" *right now*.

My sex ed teacher said that if we wanted to learn more about puberty but didn't feel comfortable asking questions, there were some books we could check out from the school or town libraries and read them on our own. She especially recommended *Are You There God? It's Me, Margaret*, by Judy Blume, for the girls in class. Of course we all rushed the school library, but I wasn't one of the lucky ones to nab a copy before they flew off the shelves. By the time I got Mom to take me to the town library, all of their copies were checked out too. Disappointed, I put my name on the waiting list, and the librarian recommended that I check out some other Judy Blume titles in the meantime.

The only one left on the shelves was called *Then Again, Maybe I Won't*. The cover was an illustration of a sparsely drawn boy, clutching a pair of binoculars. The summary on the back read:

> Ever since his father got rich from his invention and the family moved from Jersey City to a posh community on Long Island, thirteen-year-old Tony Miglione had had nothing but problems. There was his friend, Joel, who Tony knew was a shoplifter. And there was Joel's sixteen-year-old sister, Lisa, who got undressed every night without pulling down her shades. Having a lot of money brought problems, too. The new maid exiled Grandma from the kitchen, and Tony's mother was becoming a social-climbing phoney. On top of all of that, there were the growing-up problems that all boys must face. And if his parents and friends knew what Tony thought about the whole business, they'd probably flip.

I could relate to a lot of this! Well, not the "having a lot of money" part. You could absolutely describe our town as a "posh community," but my family was solidly middle-class. Other kids wore designer clothes, and their parents drove fancy cars. One of the girls in my class returned from every school break with a cinnamon honey tan and her blond hair twisted into foil-capped and plastic-beaded cornrows, and another was already going with her mother to get manicures and leg waxes. I didn't even have hair on my legs yet.

But the part about the growing-up problems resonated with me, and the girl who got undressed in front of an open window reminded me of a chapter in *Bridget's Sexual Fantasies* called "Voyeurism." I checked the book out and immediately cracked it open when I got home.

Then Again, Maybe I Won't taught me exactly what "voyeurism" meant, and what it meant for Tony. He spied on Lisa with binoculars, and sometimes when he thought about her in school he had to hold a textbook in front of his pants, and sometimes when he dreamed about her he'd have to change his bedsheets the next morning. It felt really, really good to read those parts.

I didn't try to hide this book, the way I hid my knowledge of Dad's books, because I'd gotten it from the library. It had been openly shelved; I'd openly checked it out. There should have been no shame in having it. So I left it out on my pink-and-white desk, which is where my father spotted it, and just like Tony feared his own parents would do, he went bananas.

The night Dad flipped out about *Then Again, Maybe I Won't*, he'd come into my bedroom to give me my final lights-out warning, and he saw it on my pink-and-white desk. It may have caught his attention because the title wasn't in "[Girl's Name] of [a Place]" format, and the author wasn't a woman with three names. My parents restricted my reading with the same rigor as music and movies, so I read mostly benign classics like *Anne of Green Gables* (Lucy Maud Montgomery); *Rebecca of Sunnybrook Farm* (Kate Douglas Wiggin); *A Girl of the Limberlost* (Gene Stratton-Porter); and *Julie of the Wolves* (Jean Craighead George).

Mom and Dad did allow me one guilty reading pleasure (well, as far as they knew, anyway): The Baby-Sitters Club. It's a wholesome series about a group of preteen girls who start a babysitting business and have adventures beyond child-care. There were a million of these books at the time, with candy-colored covers and a real "one of each" feel. There's one Japanese American girl (Claudia); one African American girl (Jessi); one tomboy (Kristy); one priss (Mary Anne); one diabetic (Stacey); one redhead (Mallory); and one "California girl" (Dawn), which was code for a deodorant-hating vege-tarian. There was also one boy (Logan), a Southerner who sucked.

Whenever we'd go to the bookstore, I was allowed one new BSC book. I'd start reading it on the drive home, con-tinue reading through dinner, and finish it before bedtime. Then I'd cram it into my overflowing bookshelf, which, to be fair, wouldn't have been overflowing if I'd lined up the books correctly and slid them in neatly. I was more into random piles. I didn't put *Then Again, Maybe I Won't* on my book-shelf because I didn't want a library book to get lost in this papery abyss.

I was engrossed in my latest BSC haul when Dad came in for that lights-out warning and spotted the boy with binoculars on my desk.

"What's this?" he asked, picking it up to glance at the back cover. Instantly, his face changed from casual to concerned.

"Library book," I said absentmindedly, still reading.

"Hey," Dad snapped, and he threw *Then Again, Maybe I Won't* straight at me, hard enough to knock the BSC book out of my hands. "Did you read this? Did you read this bullshit?"

The direct hit and the dirty word stunned me, and I didn't want to tell the truth, that yes, I'd read it, and yes, I had some questions about the bedsheets, but no, I'd never ask them.

Dad could tell by my face that I'd read it, that I had an inkling of what happens in a boy's underpants when he thinks about a girl in *her* underpants, and as he turned away from me in disgust he caught sight of my bookshelf, with those candy-colored books shoved in upside down and backward.

He snapped like an overstretched rubber band. In an instant, he was yanking BSC books from my bookcase and hurling them across my bedroom. One by one, they made papery slapping sounds as they hit the wall: *Kristy's Great Idea* (*THWAM!*). *Boy-Crazy Stacey* (*FFFWUP!*). *Claudia and Mean Janine* (*GWADMP!*).

Dad didn't stop there. Once all of my poor BSC books were in a defeated jumble on the floor, he turned to my Anne of Green Gables books, then the rest of the three-named lady books. I've run out of creative onomatopoeia for the smack of paper hitting drywall—just choose your own.

"Pick them up," Dad snarled when he was finally finished. "Put them back in order. None of this pigshit. Take the extra second to make things right; how many goddamned times do I have to tell you that?"

I got up, and I picked them up, and I put them back; the series in numerical order, the one-offs in alphabetical order by author's last name. I was crying too hard to ask if the three-named ladies like Louisa May Alcott should go in the M's or the A's, and I was too scared to understand the hilarity of a grown man being completely undone by a young adult book about boners.

Later, after I'd brushed my teeth and hunkered down to cry into my pillow, Dad rapped softly on the door and came in, and sat on my bed, and told me that the next time we went to the bookstore I could get two BSC books. And that was that.

Chapter 5

ALTERSPED

By seventh grade, I'd read each of Dad's sex books dozens of times. They taught me that women are supposed to make men feel good, that it's funny when fat women are naked, it's funny when fat women dress up in sexy costumes, people from different countries have sex differently, and nobody ever talks about body parts with actual body-part names. Instead, you could, and should, use cat euphemisms for the vagina, and any number of euphemisms for the penis, like:

- Egg roll
- Cannoli
- Potato
- Chopstick
- Member
- Weenie
- Sausage
- Stromboli
- Footlong
- Firecracker
- Johnson

- Pecker
- Oboe
- Trumpet
- Dong
- Lollipop

That last one still turns my face into a sour, icked-out pickle. Because the "Oral Sex" chapter of *Bridget's Sexual Fantasies* is just too much.

"I'm here to apply for the job of lollipop taster," I say.

"Oh, really?" asks Mr. Ferguson, a drab little man in his fifties. "What are your, oh, qualifications?"

"I am very fond of lollipops."

"Well then," he says, leaning forward in his chair and peering intently across the desk, "What is it that you like about sucking lollipops? Do you like the flavor, the way the cherry tastes when it firsts shoots across your buds like the explosion of a thousand brilliant suns, lighting up the galaxy of your pleasure with a fierce, radiant glow? Or the deep, sensuous essence of grape, sweet and velvet and majestic, ambrosia as it melts in your throat, intoxicating and purple?"

"Yes, all of those, all of those."

"Is it the sensation you get when you first run your tongue over its gleaming, smooth surface, feeling out all the little bumps and cavities, letting the tip of your tongue linger softly around the base, like a cow tasting sweet grass in a meadow?"

"Yes, yes," I sob, "That's it perfectly. That's just right."

"Well, then, suck my lollipop."

> He forces that thing into my mouth and as my lips close
> over it a violent sigh escapes from between his teeth, like
> steam being blown from a boiling kettle. His lollipop is
> huge, the size of a strawberry tennis ball. Now I know what
> they mean by an all-day sucker.

The accompanying photo is of a wide-eyed Bridget, gorging herself on a candy the size of a coaster. It was supposed to be funny. I probably even laughed. But, at the same time, I felt ashamed of my own squishy stomach and chubby thighs. The message was loud and clear: Skinny women were sexy; fat women were ridiculous. Skinny women deserved pleasure; fat women were undeserving of it. And, thanks to my jelly belly, and growing breasts that resembled two balls of half-risen bread dough, I saw myself in the ridiculous and undeserving camp.

Unfortunately, so did Don Wang.

Don Wang. That human snicker. He was my classmate and my tormentor, a preppy sadist who played Pop Warner football and picked on people he thought were weak. He liked to talk about girls' HANDS, wink wink, while fondling his own nipples.

I can't remember how I caught his attention, but I was one of his favorite toys. Maybe it's because I was shy, or self-conscious, or husky, or all of those things. Maybe it's because I still wore clothes and jewelry that my dad picked out for me, like those thick and pleated outlet jeans, and Formica earrings that were specifically made for, and marketed to, middle-aged women.

Don Wang seemed to live for my humiliation. I was constantly trying to do things to impress him so that maybe he'd decide I was worthy of mercy, maybe even kindness.

Nope. He decided I was worthy of the nickname "Altersped."

Our middle school's special education program was abbreviated

as "SpEd," and Don and his bland friends thought it was
hysterical to use "Sped" as a nickname for losers. I earned
"Altersped" during some merciless volleyball game in some unbearable gym class. We rotated in teams, and I was halfheartedly
shuffling toward and swatting at balls as they sailed over the
net.

"Run, Alterman!" Don guffawed as another one whizzed by
me. "Run, Sped!"

"Sara's an Altersped!" chimed in Michael Driver, another
spectacular asshole. That's maybe unfair of me, a now-adult
woman, to call a middle school boy an asshole. But he really,
really was.

"Altersped!" Don crowed and rallied the others into chanting:
"Al-ter-sped! Al-ter-sped!"

And that was that.

Don Wang never let it slide, yelling: "Altersped!" whenever
he chucked balls of paper at me in the hallway, or passed by
me on the way to the bathroom, or stuck his hands in my
lunch salads to dig out chunks of cheese and pop them into his
terrible mouth.

I didn't tell my parents about any of this because it was
embarrassing; plus, I didn't trust them not to show up at school
and split up to cover ground: Mom marching into the principal's
office; Dad marching Don Wang to the bathroom and flushing
his face down the toilet. That's just a fantasy I had. Have. Still
have. I can admit that.

Although Don Wang was an atrocious caveman, in a weird
way he did me a favor by acting as a touchstone for all the
things my parents and I were getting wrong. He made fun of my
clothes, my frizzy and product-free hair, my dangly mismatched
earrings, the fact that I didn't wear a bra, and then, the fact that I

did. One of his buddies overheard me talking about an article I'd read in *3-2-1 Contact* magazine, a children's science publication that was spun off from the TV show of the same name, and in the same media family as *Sesame Street*. That guy—whose name I can't remember but who probably had a New England douchebag name like Kent or Birch or Thatch—snickered about it to Don, and they were brutal.

"Oooh, *3-2-1 Contact*," they'd taunt. "Altersped, get me a subscription so I can be as *cool* as *you*."

That one I did admit to Dad, after I told him I didn't want to get the magazine anymore and he asked me why. He very calmly tore out the little subscription card that was attached to the middle of the magazine and handed it to me with specific instructions for what to do with it.

The next day I handed Kent/Birch/Thatch a bright red envelope that I'd found in our Christmas card stash. Inside was the subscription card with his name and his address, which I'd gotten from the school directory. He was speechless, and later I saw him tearing it up abashedly and tossing the pieces into a trash can. After that, Kent/Birch/Thatch left me alone.

It wasn't so easy with Wang, though. I started slipping off my nutty earrings on my morning bus rides to school and putting my frizzy hair up in a ponytail with the plainest scrunchies I could find. I tried ignoring him. I tried some zingy comebacks I'd read in a Lois Lowry book. I tried to disappear. When none of that worked, I tried to get him to like me. I didn't know for another few decades that if you try too hard to get people to like you, it makes you unlikable.

It didn't help my middle school reputation that I was regularly subjected to public humiliation. It also didn't help that I'd been hand-selected for the school handbell choir and was enthusiastically into it. We got to wear white cotton gloves, and ding-a-ling-dong along while our teacher, Mr. Sheen, conducted with a pencil. I liked Mr. Sheen. He was built like Santa.

Handbell choirs aren't known for being breeding grounds of popularity. But I was my best and most confident self in the music room. I could sing well and play the piano decently. I'd taught myself how to play "When the Saints Go Marching In" by ear when I was three and had been taking lessons ever since. Dad— a musician himself—loved to sit down with me so we could pick out melodies together. He once taught me the rhythm part of his absolute number one favorite song, Dave Brubeck's "Blue Rondo a la Turk." It's a plunky *dun DA, duh-DA, daaa da, dun DA, duh-DA, daaaa da*, and it made me tap my toes. I loved it.

One day in music class, some of the kids were messing around on the piano before class started. One girl played "Chopsticks," and two others played a duet of "Heart and Soul." I played the opening line of "Blue Rondo a la Turk." I knew it would blow everyone away with its, with *my*, sophistication: *dun DA, duh-DA, daaa da, dun DA, duh-DA, daaaa da*. Take *that*, Wang.

Our teacher, Mr. Sheen, perked up. "A little Brubeck, Ms. Alterman?" he said. "Not bad."

"'Blue Rondo a la Turk,'" I said proudly. "My dad taught me. It's his favorite song."

"That's not 'Blue Rondo a la Turk,'" Mr. Sheen said. "That's called 'Take Five.'"

"No," I said, my face growing hot, "it's 'Blue Rondo a la Turk.'"

"It's called 'Take Five,'" Mr. Sheen said again, kindly. "One of the most famous jazz songs of all time."

And then he played what he said was the real opening of "Blue Rondo a la Turk," a playful *BWEH-nuh, BWEH-nuh*,

*BWEH-nuh, buh-nuh-nuh, BWEH-nuh, BWEH-nuh, BWEH-
nuh, buh-nuh-nuh* that belongs in a *Peanuts* movie. I know it's
hard to transform all of these "duhs" and "bwehs" into music
in your head, so maybe just try to imagine the song that would
be playing if a panicked Charlie Brown, late for school, was
frantically running around yelling *GOOD GRIEF!!* because he
couldn't find his backpack and was going to miss his bus.

"Nice work, Altersped," Don Wang snickered.

And then he led a bunch of boys in chanting "Alter Sped! Alter
Sped!" I sank, humiliated, into a seat as Mr. Sheen distributed
sheet music for a three-part choral arrangement of "Rainbow
Connection."

That night I threw the Dave Brubeck Quartet album *Time Out*
on the turntable. If I could prove Mr. Sheen wrong in my next
music class, maybe Don Wang would apologize, or compliment
my music knowledge, or decide to ditch the Altersped.

But when I moved the needle to "Blue Rondo a la Turk"...

*BWEH-nuh, BWEH-nuh, BWEH-nuh, buh-nuh-nuh, BWEH-
nuh, BWEH-nuh, BWEH-nuh, buh-nuh-nuh.*

It was the line Mr. Sheen said was the real beginning to "Blue
Rondo a la Turk."

Suspiciously, knowingly, I moved the needle to "Take Five."

Dun DA, duh-DA, daaa da, dun DA, duh-DA, daaaa da.

The line my father had always said was "Blue Rondo a la Turk."

Dad was wrong. Wrong about his *favorite song.* That's bonkers.
It's not like when people mistake *'Scuse me while I kiss the sky* for
'Scuse me while I kiss this guy, or when my friend Marisa heard
Here come the hotstepper, I'm the lyrical gangster as *Here come the
hot pepper, I'm the leprechaun dancer.* No. This was my lifelong,
larger-than-life idol, blowing his last shred of cover.

I accused my father of being wrong, and he insisted that *I* was,

until I played "Take Five" for him on the record player. He didn't
say anything to me, just stormed out of the room.

This was the straw that shattered me. I didn't know what
to trust about my father anymore. Not his G-rated facade, not
his moods, and now, not even his knowledge of music, which
I'd taken for gospel. I went rogue in retaliation. I shoplifted a
mascara from CVS while Mom was in line at the pharmacy,
before graduating onto bigger family dress code violations, like a
mini tube skirt that I stole from T.J. Maxx. It was exhilarating.
Those were the only things I ever stole, and I snuck them to
school almost every day in my backpack. I only had the stones to
wear the skirt once, though. Still, it made me feel powerful just
to know it was in there, nestled between my Hello Kitty pencil
case and the lunch Mom packed for me, with a little love note
inside, written on a Post-it.

I also started to practice French-kissing by mashing my lips
against the eye-level soap shelf in my mom's shower. Some of
my friends practiced on their arms, but I didn't like the feeling
of kissing and being kissed at the same time, which is ridiculous,
because that's what kissing is.

All of this worked, somehow, although it wasn't Don Wang
who decided I was cool and likable. Instead, it was a boy named
Jason who sat next to me in English class. We started joking
around with each other, and soon we were partnering up for
peer-corrected language arts quizzes, and calling each other to
talk about book report assignments.

This went on for the entire second half of seventh grade,
and finally culminated in our "going out," which is in quotation
marks because every middle school relationship is in quotation
marks. We didn't "go out" anywhere. We didn't hold hands or
touch legs or even spend a single unsupervised minute together.

Our friends were always around. Plus, you think my parents
would have let me anywhere near a boy without a chaperone or
a brick wall between us? Jason asked me to a movie one time,
and my parents shut that idea down immediately. I begged and
pleaded and insisted that it wasn't, like, a date or anything. Other
kids would be there. But Mom, noticing the forbidden mascara
I'd forgotten to scrub off in the girls' bathroom before boarding
the bus home, wet a paper towel and furiously scrubbed it off
herself. Then she sent me to my room.

The last week of school was super stressful for me. Jason told
me that his family was moving to Belgium, of all places, and
I was worried that I'd never see him again, and, worse, that I
was losing my only chance at getting my first kiss. To top that
off, Mom had taken me to finally get my braces off, but the
orthodontist had opted to leave them on just my two front teeth,
for extra alignment and sensuality.

On the very last day of school, when class was dismissed for
the day and the summer, and kids tumbled out into the halls
and into each other, Jason slowed down to fall in step with me
as I walked to the bus lot. I tried my best to talk to and smile
at him with my lips closed over my bracketed bunny teeth. Outside, a row of cheerful buses sat parked on top of spray-painted
foursquare grids, waiting to ferry us away to our various parts
of town. If you dallied at the end of the day, the drivers would
honk as delicately as they could, even though they were probably
irritated, and then they'd leave you there, and you'd have to go to
the pay phone outside the principal's office and call home. They
didn't even let you use the office phone; you had to use your
own quarter.

Jason and I walked along making awkward small talk about
how much movies sucked or whatever. When we got out to the

bus lot we lingered around for a minute, sort of circling our good-byes. And then, I noticed a bunch of kids circling *us*.

"First!" a kid named Doug called out, and I didn't understand what he meant, or who he meant it for. I'd never really talked to Doug before. Doug scared me. Doug had pierced his own ear with a safety pin.

Then, *Oh god*, I thought. *He means first base.*

The bases, the sexual bases, have been loosely defined, as far as I understand. Maybe they're regional the way that East Coast "soda" is "pop" in the Midwest, "Coke" in the South, and "tonic" to my grandmother. For kids at my school, "first base" was French-kissing, "second" was feeling a girl up, "third" was feeling a girl down, and "home base" was sex. I guess that one could have been universal. There were "sloppy" versions of those things, which I thought could have involved food or technique, but I wasn't sure. Like, if you went to "sloppy third," maybe you were just bad at it, or someone found mac and cheese in your pants.

"First!" Doug called again, louder this time, and one by one the other kids in the circle joined him in chanting: "First! First! First!"

This was horrible. Sex, kissing, boy part meeting girl parts—this was all for thinking or reading about in the privacy of my bedroom. Not doing out in the open.

Jason and I looked at each other, frozen. I didn't know how to kiss anything but Mom's shower shelf. Did Jason even want to kiss me? How are you supposed to know if a boy even wants to kiss you?

And then, in a moment of sheer heroism, I leaned in toward Jason's face, pressed my lips to his, and immediately stuck my tongue completely into his mouth.

Everybody cheered. We schlurped our tongues around together,

like two fish wriggling along the surface of their tank, rooting
for food.

The whole time that Jason and I were kissing I was thinking, *Oh. My. God. This is actually happening.* The kiss lasted
either thirty seconds or thirty minutes; like preteen lips, time
is a vacuum. Then I heard an impatient bus horn honk, and I
retracted my tongue from Jason's mouth as quickly as I'd snaked
it in there. I gave him a hug that was so brief it was more like
accidentally bumping into someone, and then I ran full speed for
my bus. As I boarded, the driver gave me a funny look, and I
realized my lips were dripping. I wiped my mouth with the back
of my hand and thought: *I kissed someone!!!!!* Which quickly gave
way to: *Oh god. I hope I did it right.*

I never kissed or even saw Jason again, but I didn't care too
much. Not because he wasn't a great kid (Hi, Jason, thanks for
giving me permission to use this painfully wonderful story), but
because he was a great kid who'd served a greater purpose, even
though I didn't think about that at the time. Kissing Jason was
like loosening the bind of my parents' apron strings.

And then, in eighth grade, I met the boy who would set those
strings on fire.

Back at school, the summer after I became a Kissed Woman,
I spotted a new boy in the hallway outside homeroom. A boy
who (sorry, Jason) made me forget all other boys, forever, who
made my heart beat and my stomach hula. A boy whom I might
possibly someday kiss and then see again, or at least I hoped
I would.

A boy named Ace Casey.

Chapter 6

ACE

I learned that Ace Casey's real name was Aaron in social studies class, when our teacher, Mr. Myers, introduced him as a new kid from Pennsylvania. But he went by Ace. "Ace Casey" had the kind of cadence to it that rolled right off the tongue, and I wanted his tongue to roll right over me. It was the first time I can remember having a thought like that, and every time I thought about him, my face flushed into that color that cinnamon tastes like.

Ace Casey had fauxhawked blond hair that badly wanted to curl, and an anarchy pin on the outside pocket of his backpack. He was a few inches shorter than me, and he pursed his lips like a superspy with secrets.

Mr. Myers placed him three seats behind me, and as he passed by my desk I could smell his cologne. It smelled like the woods, and I recognized the brand because I'd sniffed a sample of it in the pages of a magazine.

Mr. Myers was a big fan of anonymous surveys, and he often asked the kids sitting in the front row to take out a piece of paper, write down their birthday or favorite food or career aspiration, and pass it back so the kids in the second row could do the same, and so on. Then he collected all of the papers. I can't remember what he did with them, if anything at all. He may have been killing time before the end-of-the-period buzzer buzzed and we all moved on to become some other teacher's problem.

So Ace sat three seats behind me, and even a week into his presence I could tell he was a heavy metal fan because beneath his unbuttoned flannels with the sleeves rolled up, he wore black T-shirts with angry-looking logos. I didn't know much about heavy metal, but I *did* know that angry-looking logos, with sharp typeface and skulls, lightning bolts, et cetera, were typical traits of heavy metal band T-shirts. And I knew about exactly one such band, Megadeth, because I'd overheard some of the high-intensity alterna-kids on the bus talking about Dave Mustaine's sick guitar licks.

I didn't know how to broadcast that I knew about Megadeth. There was no way in hopscotch that my mother would have bought me a Megadeth T-shirt, much less one of their albums. But I wanted Ace to look at me, to *see* me—the girl with the wonky self-made French braid and the terrible nickname—and to want to see me more.

Then one afternoon Mr. Myers said: "Okay, front row. Take out a piece of paper, write down your favorite singer or band, and pass it back." He spoke with a thick slab of Massachusetts accent. *Paypah. Singah.*

Front row! That was me! It was me every day, but that day felt like *the* day. I tore a fresh page from my Lisa Frank psychedelic unicorn notebook and wrote "Megadeath." Well, didn't just write it but *drew* it to the best of my ability, re-creating the angles and fangs of the logo I'd memorized by staring at Ace's chest at every opportunity. My drawing didn't look quite right—I realized later that I'd spelled it wrong, writing *death* instead of *deth*. Hell. Damn. But I was pleased with my own clever plan to catch Ace

Casey's attention, even after I passed the paper behind me to Don Wang and he snickered: "Altersped."

I wanted to die and do the whole world a favor by taking a bleeding and begging Don Wang with me to the other side. But if Ace heard, he didn't let on.

And anyway, the Megadeth plot flopped like a Frenching tongue. Ace Casey and I didn't speak a word to each other. I had a massive, sweaty crush on him for the next two years, until sophomore year of high school, when by chance we sat next to each other in Spanish class.

Our Spanish classroom was set up with long tables in a U shape around the perimeter of the room, "to facilitate engaging conversation *en español*," my syllabus said. Every language class in school was totally immersive. I assume that kids taking Latin were just lobbing legal terms and Gregorian chants at each other all the time.

Dad was mildly outraged about the whole thing. "How the hell do they think you're going to speak a language that you don't speak?" he'd grumbled over dinner when I told him. "That's absurd."

It was absurd, but I didn't mind, because I got to not-speak a language at a shared table where my leg occasionally accidentally on purpose brushed up against Ace Casey's. He wore a wallet chain sometimes, and when I wore a dress I could feel the cool metal links make soft imprints in my exposed flesh. I wore dresses a lot. By then it was the grunge era of fashion, so instead of wiggling into mini tube skirts, I preferred long babydoll dresses with flannel shirts tied strategically around my waist. Mom and Dad were fine with this. They bought me a bunch of modest dresses—"Totally funky!" Mom called them—and let me wear them with Doc Martens, or Birkenstock sandals. If I wiggled in my classroom chair *just so*, I could casually hike the hem of my long dresses up to expose my legs, which, unbeknownst to my mom, I'd begun to shave, even above the knee.

I couldn't bring myself to speak to Ace out loud, maybe because I was insecure, or intimidated, or didn't yet know the Spanish for *Please take my body somewhere and have at it.* That may not even translate. It felt completely unnatural to want a real person like this. I was mortified by my own lust.

But one day we started scribbling little notes to each other in my notebook, at first banal stuff, like "Did you do the homework?" or "What's our homework?" or "Fuck homework."

Soon we were sharing a page, covertly writing movie quotes and song lyrics that captured our moods. I still have our notes. Here's one:

Me:
Ace-ito,
Freshmen are fun to step on. They make a neato sound. "Help me! Help me! I'll give you money!" It's kind of cool to have power. Yeah.

Ace:
One time I had a cat who liked to meow, except he made a sound like this: "Eee! Eee!" So I said, "Gee, Mr. Cat! You sure like the letter E!" Then he scratched my face and I almost bled to death. Good thing I fell on top of him and crushed his skull. I had a hamster once, too.

Me:
My mom had a friend who liked cats. Her cat used to sleep in the clothes dryer. His name was Mr. Fuzzy. One time, Mr. Fuzzy was sleeping in the dryer, but my mom's

friend didn't see him. So she started the dryer so she could have toasty warm clothes. "Mrrrrrreeeooowwww!!!" Mr. Fuzzy is now named "Mr. Burned to a Crisp and Deteriorated." Isn't that a funny story?

Ace:

I would never try to eat a cat unless it tried to eat me first.

I used to watch TV a lot. One time I was eating some fish and I laughed and it flew out of my mouth into the bathtub! I figured it was happier there, swimming in the suds, except now I can't take a shower at all, and I'm all smelly! I don't eat fish anymore because what if it fell in the john? Cows.

And then he drew me a little picture of a cross-eyed cow.

Ace wrote his lowercase letter "a" like a typewriter did, like a lowercase letter "d" that had given up. I practiced that "a" in the back of my notebook the way some girls practiced their first name with the last name of their crushes, as their names might appear once married, if name-changing were important to them. I didn't change my name when I got married. I *did* change my lowercase "a" to match Ace Casey's, maybe so he'd see it on the page and decide we were a natural fit, which is what the failed Megadeth incident was supposed to accomplish.

Luckily, happily, we were paired up for a team project about Mexican culture by our teacher, Señora Wilkins. *La diabla.* She was mean as hell. But when she announced the project partners, I wanted to kiss her. No tongue.

Ace and I decided to bake something for our project, for some reason. It might have been my mom who suggested it. I think she thought I would bring this random boy over to our house so she could keep an eye on us in the kitchen for the however many hours it took to make Mexican pastries. But then, by beautiful chance again, our oven broke. I had to go to Ace's house.

My parents were terrified that Ace's parents wouldn't be home, so I assured them that, yes, his mother would be with us in the kitchen the entire time, an assurance that I had absolutely no business making and turned out to be wrong anyway. Ace's mom wasn't home. We were blissfully, awkwardly alone.

I accidentally picked a complicated recipe for *pan dulce*, with a million steps and two separate rise times, which meant we had hours of just sitting around, waiting for yeasted dough to puff up. It was almost for sure an accident—I wasn't savvy enough to be calculating; plus, Ace and I really communicated only through those notes. The idea of having to actually speak out loud scared me more than middle school gym-class volleyball games.

We measured and mixed in silence, mostly, while an Alice in Chains CD growled softly in the background. I tried to flirt with him as well as any girl wearing discount corduroys can manage. Then the dough had to sit under a warm, damp cloth for forty-five minutes.

He swaddled it with care, then when he asked if I wanted to see his room, I practically choked on my own drool, or maybe it was the cloud of flour I'd just clapped into his face, trying to be whimsical.

"Cool," I said, as casual as a foghorn.

Ace Casey's second-floor bedroom was a mall goth's wet dream. His bed had black sheets and a maroon comforter, and was positioned under the watchful eye of a massive Metallica poster taped to the ceiling. A dog-eared copy of *A Nietzsche Reader* sat casually on his nightstand. A black electric guitar stood at attention in a stand next to the bed. I could practically smell the heady musk of Ace Casey's brooding.

To the left of his double bed was a walk-in closet; to the right, a window that opened out onto the flat roof of the screened-in porch off the kitchen. Ace stepped out of the window onto the roof of the porch, and then turned back to offer me his hand. I took it and stepped through, and from there we scrambled up the steep roof of the main part of the house. You could see the whole neighborhood from up there, but of course all I could focus on was his edible neck.

Who knows what we were talking about. Spanish homework, maybe, or quoting our favorite lines from *The Princess Bride*. I just remember sitting beside him, breathing in the oily scent of tar roof tiles and the musk of his cologne, silently calculating how close I could come to pressing my outstretched leg against his before it got weird. It was different in class, with no room to spread out; our limbs, crammed and cramped between table legs and backpacks, touching out of necessity.

And then he kissed me. No tongue. Who cares.

I will remember the feel of Ace Casey's lips for the rest of my life. Soft and confident, a little bit cold. He kissed the way he carried himself. After a minute he tried to pull me on top of him, but I held back. I didn't want him to feel how heavy I was.

That evening, after the *pan dulce* was finished, I called home for a ride, and when my dad showed up he shook Ace's hand and said, "He has a mohawk." Said it *to* him.

Dad and I were both quiet on the ride home. I was recovering from the humiliation of Dad's mohawk comment. Dad must have been thinking about how much trouble this mohawked "study buddy" could be for his daughter.

I was only fifteen, and still a year away from being allowed to date. Ace and I met up at his house again to work on the poster for our Spanish project, and to kiss for a while. We got an A on our presentation, and he asked me to be his girlfriend. I said yes without even taking a second to breathe, and figured I'd work out a way for us to see each other.

Obviously, I made up a lot of lies about a lot of Spanish projects. Ace's family had a computer and modem, so I'd just tell my parents that we needed to dial up the server at school to get homework assignments. In hindsight, this lie was paper-thin. It's true that by the mid '90s our school did have a server that was connected to four phone lines, so only four people could access the server at a time. (To this day, I do not understand a single thing about how that worked. Explanation pending from my old-school tech-savvier friends.) But so few people had modems at the time, posting assignments online would have been pointless.

We snuck around for a while, and then a year later, on my sixteenth birthday, I outed myself to my parents as having a boyfriend. They just looked at each other, and it was clear that they already suspected, even knew. After that, I wasn't allowed to go over to Ace's house unless his mother confirmed that she'd be home.

Ace and I quickly became inseparable. We wrote each other earnest poems and beautiful letters and he made mixtapes of German industrial metal and EDM for me, and when I clutched his dry, calm palm under that table in Spanish class I felt sure of my place in the world, or at least of my place in high school. He had his own phone number—not a separate line but a unique ring—and I used the last four digits as my ATM pin, my locker combination, the code name for "Ace" in my diary. I liked the feeling of using something uniquely his to protect something uniquely mine. He brought flowers to my choir concerts and stormed out of my junior year production of *Guys and Dolls* because I had to kiss another guy, and it was too painful for him to watch.

We were slow and steady when it came to rounding the proverbial bases. We didn't have a lot of time alone together, and anyway, I felt paralyzed by the fat-shaming from my dad's books and harbored a ton of hang-ups about the rolls of stomach fat that stacked like a layer cake whenever I sat down.

Maybe worst of all, I thought I was just supposed to be making Ace feel good, with no clue about how to ask for my own pleasure, or that it was even an option. Kissing Ace, holding his hand in class, feeling his arm around my shoulders as we walked the hallways—for me, that was hitting the pleasure ceiling. When I wrote that I instantly imagined Bridget in a small glass room, too tall to fully stand.

I had no idea *how* to make Ace feel good and was terrified that he'd laugh with his friends about my clumsy hands and mouth, or dump me for a more experienced girl, or both. Until one day in the den, as I was watching a nature documentary with my parents, it hit me: I had the books.

That's how Bridget became my personal sexual sensei, and all of the official *Sex Manual* books became my official how-to guides for pleasing my man. Any time I was alone in the house, I'd snatch one of the books and race with it up to my bedroom, hunkering down in my closet so if my parents came in I could quickly stuff it under a pile of shoes. I took copious notes on oral sex, bondage, S and M, rape fantasies, tickle fantasies, elevator fantasies, the best way to peel an Irishman's potato. I took it all very seriously, and sincerely—even the dated language and ideals—and learned how to talk about sex, even during sex, like it was the late 1970s.

The first time Ace showed me his lollipop, I was scared, but ready. *Just let the tip of your tongue linger softly around the base,* I thought, trying to remember verbatim how Bridget aced her job interview at the sucker factory. *Just stuff the whole thing in and widen your eyes like you're loving it.* About forty-five seconds after I started, I made the disappointing discovery that what comes out of a lollipop does not taste like candy.

Bridget's dedication to costumes really rang true for me. I was a theater kid, and I liked Halloween. I still had a box of dress-up clothes in the basement that had been updated as recently as the tenth grade. Maybe if I dressed up in a costume and reenacted some of the chapters from *Bridget's Sexual Fantasies,* I'd be more confident about, and better at, sex stuff.

So I saved up my babysitting and dog-walking money, and blushed my way through a garter belt debacle at Victoria's Secret in the Natick Mall. I just wanted to get in and out at lightning speed, so I snatched a black lace garter belt with matching stockings, picked up a few pairs of underpants with ruffled rears, and hustled up to the counter with my head ducked down, just in case anyone from school or, worse, any of my mom's friends happened to be shopping there.

The bored-looking employee at the register looked me up and down. "Where's your bra?" she asked, snapping a gob of pink gum.

"My, um, my what?" I asked, barely above a whisper.

She rolled her eyes. "Your *bra,*" she said, and pointed to a sign announcing a promotion: "Free bra with any purchase of $40 or more."

"No thanks," I mumbled. "I don't want one."

"What do you mean you don't want a free bra? It's a *free bra,*" Gum Face said, incredulous and clueless about my growing humiliation. Scratch that—she probably just didn't notice, or care.

"I just want to buy this stuff, please," I said, and she closed her eyes and sighed.

"I don't know how I'm going to ring you up if you don't get the bra," she said. "The system won't ring up a sale over $40 if I don't scan a tag for a bra. Marleen!" she called across the store.

A voice called back from somewhere over by the pajamas. "Yeah?"

"She doesn't want her bra!"

"Who doesn't?"

"This girl. She got a garter belt and accessories but doesn't want the free bra."

"Why doesn't she want the bra? It's a *free bra*."

Gum Face turned to me. "Why don't you want the free bra?"

"Fine!" I said. "Fine. I'll get the bra." And I scrambled, lava-cheeked, over to the push-up bra section, picked out a simple black one, and raced back to the counter. A line had formed in my absence. Women carrying sensible purses and clutching satin nightgowns were leering at me. Girls in soccer uniforms with fistfuls of cotton briefs were giggling. "There," I said to Gum Face, throwing it down on the counter. "Can you please ring me up now?"

I paid cash for all of it; the babysitting money, the dog-walking money, plus $20 that some relative had sent for my birthday. Then I got the h-e-double hockey sticks out of there.

Unfortunately, instead of feeling sexy and confident in the garter belt, I felt stupid. According to Bridget, Ace and I should be trussing each other up like turkeys or riding each other like rodeo bulls or pretending he was a tennis instructor helping me to perfect my grip. But often we were so confused by whatever knots we were supposed to be tying or talk we were supposed to be talk-ing, that we just gave up and watched a movie. Usually *Aliens*.

Where were his parents? Who can remember. Ace had two older brothers who were around only during their college breaks. I think Mr. Casey worked late and Mrs. Casey was deeply involved with the local League of Women Voters.

My parents did everything they could to keep my relationship with Ace innocent. They gave us cheesy theater tickets and made us go with them to U-pick apple orchards. If I went to Ace's house on a weekend, my mom would always call over to talk to his parents while I was there, but if nobody answered the phone? *Ding-dong*, the doorbell would ring and there would be Dad, come to "surprise" me and Ace by taking us out to a "family dinner" at an Italian place nearby. It was humiliating. And confusing too. Why not just drag me home if he didn't want me to be alone with my boyfriend, instead of dragging us both out to a restaurant? Maybe Dad enjoyed the sadism of watching a nervous teenage boy sweat into a bowl of ravioli.

Despite all of that, they liked Ace. He was enrolled in all of our school's AP classes and was an A student. Even though he dressed like a punk rocker he was a bashful marshmallow, or at least could behave like one in front of adults. I don't think my parents objected to Ace Casey as much as they objected to the idea of my having a boyfriend.

I loved him. Crazy love. I wanted to eat him alive, suck the marrow from his bones. We dated for a year and a half, I think? Two years? A month feels like a year when you're in high school. To commemorate our one-year anniversary, my father bought the two of us matching motorcycle jackets. I was thrilled, because it meant that Ace was finally and fully Dad-approved. Plus, I thought the jackets were super cool, until the look on Ace's face told me that they were not cool, and that this kind of thing was not cool in general. Disappointed, I shoved mine into the back of my closet, and never told Ace that I was hoping we could wear them out together, like a couple of greaser lovebirds who couldn't wait to pin each other.

I made Ace take me to prom. He was practically kicking and screaming at the "establishment" of it all. In protest he wore combat boots with his tuxedo. It was miserable. Ace wouldn't dance with me, just sat outside and sulked on the porch of the snooty, stupid country club our school had booked for the affair. Afterward, we drove to a soccer field in Ace's boxy black Pontiac and I gave him an angry hand job, still wearing the black polyester opera gloves I'd bought to go with my dress. When that was over, he apologized and said he'd just wanted to be alone with me all night, not doing the Macarena with a bunch of preppy fools. I caved, then we slow-danced under the stars while his car stereo blasted a Rammstein song. I was wearing tall platform heels, and I could practically rest my chin on top of his soft, blond head.

A few months after prom Ace and I had sex for the first time: in his bedroom, by candlelight, on top of a worn pink towel, to a special mixtape he'd made of Metallica songs. Between that and Ace's Metallica ceiling poster, it was a fully immersive James Hetfield experience.

Given that sex was swathed in shame and repression in my house, it's surprising that I didn't feel nervous or guilty leading up to the big event. There was a little anxiety about whether it was going to hurt, whether we were going to get caught. We decided to double up on the birth control, so Ace bought condoms; I was already on the pill.

That might sound surprising, given all I've laid out about my parents and their wholesome world. But when I was fifteen, I'd awoken in the middle of the night in excruciating pain— it felt like something in my abdomen was going to detonate. I managed to stumble to my parents' room, and my dad drove me to the emergency room.

A triage nurse took my vitals, helped me change into a hospital gown, and said she was going to take me down to the radiology department for some imaging tests.

"Is there any chance you could be pregnant?" she'd asked.

Before I could answer, Dad cut in. "There'd better not be," he said, and although he tried to sound like he was joking, I could tell that he meant it. I could tell that he actually had no idea whether or not his teenage daughter could be pregnant.

The hospital ran some tests, the nurse pulled my dad aside for a long chat, and then they sent me home with a bottle of pain medication and no explanation of what was going on.

"So," Dad said on the drive, "good news. It's not your appendix or anything like that. It's...um..."

As I watched my father struggle to come up with the right words, I started to panic. *Cancer*, I thought. *It has to be cancer. Why else would he be this freaked out? It has to be—* "It's the dreaded *ovulation*," Dad blurted, and he turned bright red. "Well, no. It's...uh...a cyst of some kind. On your ovaries. And when you ovulated, it ruptured. I think. Let your mother explain it to you when we get home."

That was the closest thing to a "sex talk" that my father and I ever had. On the way home, we had to stop at a 24-hour pharmacy so Dad could fill a prescription for a medication that would drastically reduce my risk of ovarian cysts: hormonal birth control.

Who was my prudish, porno-writing dad to argue with this irony? Doctor's orders.

I know it made him uncomfortable in general that his daughter was on the pill. But once it was clear that Ace and I were dating, and there was a real threat that I'd put those birth control pills to *work*, well, I can't imagine the distress that must have caused him.

After Ace and I had sex he grew distant, then, dickish. It seems so obvious now. We had sex only two more times, both in the middle of the day when the sunlight was bright and I could see his face. See how his mind was somewhere else.

After we were finished the third time, the last time, I put my head on Ace's chest to listen to his heartbeat, and when I looked up at his beautiful face, he was smiling blissfully at the ceiling.

"What are you thinking about?" I asked softly, happily, hoping he'd murmur something into my ear about how beautiful I was, or how lucky he was, or how much he loved me.

But he snarfed, and said, "Hard-on did something hilarious in math today." "Hard-on" was Ace's best friend, Chris Hardy. "He was just, like, quoting *No Exit* in a Beavis voice. Like, 'Huh-huh. Hell is other people! Huh-huh.' It was fucking hilarious."

Ace Casey broke my heart over the phone. I called him to plan a movie night, and we fought over what to see. I wanted *Evita* and he wanted *The People vs. Larry Flynt*, ew, or *Beavis and Butt-Head Do America*, obviously.

I caved. "Fine, fine," I said. "Saturday or Sunday? What time?"

"Actually...um...," he said, and let it hang for what felt like a million years. And then I knew what was coming. I could feel it.

"You're breaking up with me," I said, and that hung for a million years more.

He never said it. The next morning I found a note in my locker. The gist of it was that it wasn't me, it was him, that he needed to figure some things out, that he would always love me.

A few weeks later, I caught Ace Casey gently, passionately

kissing a goth girl outside the door to the music room as I left concert choir rehearsal. I knew exactly who she was. She'd once threatened to kick my ass in a bathroom by the auditorium because I'd coughed indignantly in the general direction of her clove cigarette. *You're not supposed to smoke in the bathroom, Abigail.*

And that was it. I was destroyed and spent several weeks skipping after-school choir practices to drive around alone until curfew, listening to Jewel's "Foolish Games" on repeat and crying into spicy chicken sandwiches from the Wendy's drive-through. At night I would crawl into my parents' bed, and Mom would wrap her arms around me while Dad relocated to my bed. He said he liked sleeping in there anyway because he could count the glow-in-the-dark stars on my ceiling, instead of sheep.

Somehow I got through the rest of the school year, got through Ace and Abigail's showy makeouts and the day they decided to ironically dress up in preppy clothes to troll the lacrosse kids. I made it through watching them slow-dance in a mediocre hotel ballroom at senior prom and sobbing in the bathroom about what an extra traitor he was for dancing with her, a year after refusing to dance with me. I made it to and through graduation, and then I went to college in New York and tried to move on with a boy who had stringy hair and a guitar in his room, which he was unable to play.

I don't remember who started it, but during my second semester of college, Ace and I began writing emails to each other. At first detached, generic catch-up notes, then cryptic poems, then more graphic stuff that I mistook for romantic declarations. During spring break we met up and made out. It happened again over the summer. Then, winter break. And so on, until we graduated from college, and I moved to Myrtle Beach to bartend at an Applebee's and be an aimless chain-smoking asshole. Ace stayed in Boston.

Every time I went home to visit my parents, I'd shoot him an email or a text to meet up. Once, we slipped into historic Walden Pond to skinny-dip among transcendental vibes and toxic algae. Night swimming there was illegal, and we had to park half a mile away and tiptoe through the woods, so that any patrolling local cops wouldn't catch and ticket us for being reckless idiots.

Myrtle Beach was all wrong for me, and it was miserable. Dad flew down to pack up my stuff with me, and then drove solo for fifteen hours in a rented moving truck while I drove my own car, then promptly, humbly, moved into my parents' basement. Once I'd settled back in Massachusetts I was hopeful that Ace and I would reconnect for real and for good, but he moved abroad, to Berlin. We'd still see each other once or twice a year, make out again, go away again. And so on, and so on, for ten fucking years.

It, and I, was so pathetic. But I loved him so deeply, and I truly, stupidly thought that Ace still loved me too. Why else would we keep returning to each other like this? It was mostly just kissing, though, which is absurd, right? Ten years of kissing somebody? I should have picked up on how weird that was, I guess. These makeouts would always end with me crying about how we were meant to be together, and he would kind of nod and then kind of slip away.

When we were in our mid-twenties, after I'd finally emotionally excavated myself from the basement and gotten a proper apartment, Ace was home for a visit, so we met up for drinks in Boston. I had too much whiskey and pushed him to tell me why he'd fallen in love with me in high school, and he said he couldn't remember.

Later that night, when we were making out, I felt him playfully snap the waistband of my underwear, and then he laughed.

"What is it?" I asked, giggling, sure that I was in on the joke.

"Large." He chuckled, and tugged on the tag.

I rolled off of him and curled up into a ball on the edge of my bed, wondering if he'd always laughed at my body. Ace just shrugged and rolled over to the other side of my bed to check his phone.

After a few minutes the antiseptic sting of humiliation began to wear off, and I realized that I didn't know, or love, this person. I drove him to the subway and sent him off forever into the underground.

I've heard he's a DJ now.

I've heard Don Wang has daughters now.

Chapter 7

OUT OF THE WOODS

My parents nearly met a million times, before they finally did.

In the mid-1970s, my mother was working as the receptionist for the Boston Celtics, and on the weekends she had a second job running the mail-order division for a company that made sports yearbooks. Dad was working for a weekly newspaper. He'd gone to college for journalism and had wanted to be a reporter but was able to land jobs only in production departments, organizing and arranging what other people wrote.

Mom liked the solitude of her second job. The sports yearbook company's office building was a ghost town on the weekends, and she liked having the building to herself. One quiet Saturday she was head-down in an order, when out of nowhere she heard, "I'm going out for a sandwich, do you want one?"

Mom jerked her head up to find an impeccably dressed and generously sideburned man standing in her office doorway. It was my dad, of course. One of the printers his newspaper used was located in the same building. The presence of a cute stranger startled Mom into a full horse-on-roller-skates situation, and by the time she recovered from the fluster, he was gone. A few months passed and she forgot about him, but then winter rolled around and the sideburns showed up again, this time with a haircut and a filthy mitten he'd found in a pile of snish. "Snish" is a made-up Massachusetts word, coined by the legendary Boston weatherman Dick Albert, to describe a cocktail of snow and slush.

"Is this yours?" the tall drink of muttonchops asked my mom, and when she replied that no, it certainly wasn't, he said, "Oh. Well, then would you like to go out with me tomorrow?"

She would.

They went to see *The Pink Panther Strikes Again* and then to a deli, where my atheist Jewish father tried to convince his shiksa date to split a tongue sandwich.

She would not.

But she married him two years later. I wanted a love story like theirs.

Around the time my parents met, there was a huge and hot music spot in Boston's Kenmore Square, where the trumpet player was notorious for choosing a woman from the crowd, hoisting her up onto his shoulders, and parading around the room, *brrh brrh barurrhh*-ing merrily along. One fateful, unforgettable night, he chose my mom.

"I was wearing all purple," she told me. "And the trumpet guy must have noticed because of that. I was mortified. I kept saying, 'No, no, put me down!' But he just carried on and carried me all around."

Dad loved that story, because he was there.

This was years before the filthy snish mitten incident, before he noticed my cute mother typing away alone on a Saturday.

"I'll never forget it," he said, "this long-haired woman all in purple. She was trying to laugh, but you could tell she did not want that putz carrying her around."

They figured out this near-miss on one of their early dates and discovered several more: They'd once lived a few miles from each other in tiny seaside towns on the North Shore, and again in Central Massachusetts, where my father would take back roads to get to work, and drive right past my mother's house. They were in England at the same time as teenagers, when Mom was working as a nanny and Dad was backpacking/cavorting around with his best friend.

I love the inevitability of my parents' marriage, how their lives crisscrossed for years before intertwining for good, how they unknowingly shared a history. Their courtship feels peppered with the same quirky whimsy that defined my childhood: the birthday cakes, the road-trip games, the cupcake tea parties that Mom catered for me and my dolls, the pop-up greeting cards Dad sent me at summer sleepover camp.

My parents' relationship shaped my idea of how a love story should begin. How, when you're meant to be with someone, you'll find each other. I guess I had such a hard time giving up on Ace Casey because I'd seen our relationship as having that rare and special serendipity to it. I know now that there's not a ton of serendipity to sitting next to someone in a high school class, or whimsy in eating the same limp french fries in the same high school cafeteria.

And yet, I married someone from high school.

In early 2007, at a music club in Boston near Kenmore Square, I met a clean-cut guy in a button-down shirt while I was standing on my tiptoes and waving a twenty-dollar bill, trying to get the bartender's attention. I felt a tap on my shoulder, and when I spun around, there was a guy with perfect teeth and rolled-up sleeves, holding his hand out for me to shake.

"Hi!" he said, with a smile brighter than the stage lighting. "I'm Sam."

No man in a bar had ever offered me a handshake before. Had any man in a bar ever offered any woman a handshake before? It doesn't matter. I took his hand, and then I recognized him, from ye olde 01776.

Sam and I went to the same elementary, middle, and high schools, but we hadn't known each other. I was one year ahead of him, and besides that, while he'd been in the Outdoors Club and taken all of the AP classes, I'd had an indoor sensibility and barely did homework. Still, he looked vaguely familiar, and we quickly figured out that his father's house was across the street from one of my friends. Sam's next-door neighbors had an aging, netless tennis court in their yard, and they didn't mind if kids rode their bikes around in there. I'd played in that tennis court a lot. Sam had too.

Chatting at the bar that night, Sam and I remembered that we'd been in touch years prior, through an early social media platform that let you connect with other users based on the people and places you had in common. He'd sent me a coy message out of nowhere, I'd playfully accused him of flirting, and that was that. A few years after that, he saw a coworker reading a piece I wrote for a local newspaper, and told her, "I know her!" And the coworker said, "Me too!" because it was my friend Rachel.

That night we shook hands, the night that our lives finally crisscrossed in person, all of the other showgoers melted into the background as I hit it off with this hometown guy who, as we discovered, now lived just over a mile from me. We often went to the same neighborhood Irish bar for Tuesday night trivia. *This* was the stuff of serendipity.

"Maybe we should...go together?" I asked.

Sam put my number into his phone and promised to call. I went home that night and looked him up in my senior yearbook.

I found him in a photo of the Outdoors Club, taken in a lecture hall next to the music room. He was standing almost directly behind where I'd stood, possibly on the same day, for a photo with the concert choir.

The following Tuesday we met up for trivia. I wore an olive-green Guinness T-shirt and brought my giant red dog, Murphy, which was all maybe too on the nose for an Irish bar. Sam wore another button-down shirt and turned out to be a major asset in the music category.

I learned that he worked for a software company, was close with his family, played in a flag football league, and mentored a little boy through Big Brothers Big Sisters of America. He briefly squeezed my knee and said "Amazing!" after I nailed a question about *Pee-wee's Playhouse*.

While we waited for the trivia overlord to tally scores for a round about movie posters, Sam talked about his love for the woods and mountains. He was an experienced and passionate backpacker who had started hiking with his mom when he was nine. In the summers he'd go up to New Hampshire for programs with the Appalachian Mountain Club, including a two-week camp called AMC Teen Adventures, for which he wandered around the White Mountains doing Sisyphean tasks like moving giant rocks onto or off of sections of the Appalachian Trail.

"I wore my AMC Teen Adventures T-shirt on my first day at college!" he said. He went to Bates, which seems like a place for woods-and-mountain people, or at least for people who own woods- and mountain-specific footwear. A place where an AMC Teen Adventures T-shirt probably gets you laid.

"Maybe we should go together," he said, echoing my casual trivia invitation.

I wasn't sure if he was serious, or just making that flighty kind of offer that gets you out of a surprise conversation quickly, like when you bump into someone you haven't seen in a long time and don't really want to see again. "Great to see you! We should *totally* hang out sometime!" and then you part ways without making any actual plans.

Even if he was serious, I didn't mind. I really wanted to spend more time with Sam, who talked about backpacking the way a hungry person might recall their favorite meal. Maybe it's crazy to sign yourself up for alone time in the woods with someone you've technically met only twice, but we shared a hometown and a history. It put me at ease and reminded me of my parents' story.

Besides, I loved camping: driving around until you find, and claim, the perfect site; overstuffing a tent with queen-sized air mattresses and down comforters; making s'mores by a roaring fire; and then driving back out for pizza or to check out a multi-media art installation exhibit at a local museum. That's the kind of camping I did many times with high school friends. Never family, though. I once tried to convince my parents to go, but Dad visibly shuddered at the thought.

"No way, José," he'd said. "People shouldn't sleep in the woods. It's why God made hotels."

"I thought you didn't believe in God?" I asked.

"Hotels are the only proof that God exists," he said.

That trivia night gave way to more trivia nights, and movies, and dinners, and, after just a month of dating, Sam planned a three-day trip for us to backpack and camp along one of his favorite routes in New Hampshire. He took me to a huge REI to buy rain gear because, he said, the weather in the White Mountains is notoriously unpredictable, even in the summertime.

"My first job was at REI," he told me proudly, and pulled a weathered paper card from his wallet. "When I was seventeen I got hired as a sales associate at a new store in Framingham before it opened, and I got to do really cool training on all of the gear, help set up the store, and build all of the merchandise displays. *And* I had an employee discount. It was the greatest."

Watching a grown man get so excited about his high school job was, well, adorable. In high school I was a hostess at a mediocre Italian restaurant, where I made minimum wage, endured a cartoonishly evil manager, and learned from the Brazilian line cooks how to say "Blow me" in Portuguese.

"I still know my employee ID number," Sam said, smiling. "It was 68521. My best friend Josh was 68523. I was two better than him."

"I don't suppose you get, like, an employee emeritus discount?" I asked, eyeing the sales racks and already dreading the inevitable declined transaction on my debit card. At that point in my life, I was usually teetering on the brink of an overdraft. But Sam zipped me into a full-priced anorak the color of a baby lizard. He tightened the hood around my face, kissed me on the nose, and said, "You look so cute!" Then he bought it for me. He offered to buy matching waterproof rain pants, but I declined, because they made me feel dorky.

Sam did all of the planning and packing for the trip. I brought dinner over to his apartment the night before we left, and he had what looked like an entire REI's worth of gear spread out all over his living room, including a little camping percolator so I could have coffee. Sam hated coffee and teased me constantly about my addiction to what he called bitter brown trash water. He'd bought this little percolator just for me.

He was also bringing two sleeping bags that could zip together into one large nest. "For extra body heat," he said, and I took that as a *sexy* sign I wouldn't need to bring pajamas. "They're made of down," he said apologetically, "but as long as nothing gets wet, it should be fine."

"Are you kidding?" I asked. "What's better than snuggling in a tent?"

The next morning I returned to Sam's apartment with all of *my* camping supplies: a plastic shopping bag containing my new raincoat, two cotton tank tops, two pairs of underwear, one extra pair of socks, some toiletries, and a half batch of brownies I baked as a surprise. Sam had told me to pack light, so I figured I'd wear the same pair of Old Navy cotton cargo pants for all three days of hiking, and never wear pants at night. Wink.

I was late, and Sam was eager to get on the road for the two-plus-hour drive to the trailhead up in Franconia, so he quickly shoved my stuff into a backpack without looking at it. The back-pack surprised me. The only one I owned, and maybe had ever owned, was left over from middle school: a black L.L.Bean book bag with my initials monogrammed in white. The same one I used to sneak contraband miniskirts and mascara.

The pack Sam handed to me was the length of my torso, with a thick, padded belt that he said would take the weight off of my shoulders. He wrapped and buckled it around my hips and yanked the adjustable strap until it felt like the good-bye hug I got from a surfer who dumped me at a Bugaboo Creek Steak-house but still, like, really wanted to be in my life because of my incredible heart.

"Oh wow, it's, um, heavy," I said, trying to sound less panicked and more observational, like, *Oh wow, it's made of fabric.*

On the drive to Franconia, Sam told me all about the

itinerary he'd planned for us. We'd hike up a mountain to the summit, break for snacks, continue along a ridge, eat lunch on a *different* mountain summit, then make our way 4 miles down *that* mountain to our campsite. It would be 8.5 miles total.

"And that's all...today?" I asked, thinking, *Fuck. Don't panic. Fuck. Fuck.*

"Yup," Sam said. "We'll go nice and slow, probably about a mile, mile and a half an hour. I brought you some special snacks. We can have them while we look at all the nice views."

Those nice views were bullshit. It started drizzling about two hours into our excruciating uphill climb, and I couldn't see a thing beyond my own damp boots.

At first it was kind of romantic, the rain making poetic little patter sounds across the spiky foliage canopy of coniferous trees. I knew they were coniferous trees because from the moment we set foot in the woods, Sam offered up little factoids, like "See the beeches and maples? This is a hardwood forest," or "Smell the spruce? We're getting into boreal forest territory," or "This whole mountain is a spectrum of microclimates!"

I made sure Sam was watching when I pulled on my new raincoat, so he'd be reminded of how adorable my little hooded face was.

After an hour, it stopped raining. Because it started hailing. By the time we reached the snack summit, the sky was pelting us with icy pellets the size of nickels. Every strike on the back of my exposed calves felt like a razor nick.

The summit was all thin fog and loose rock, with a narrow ridge trail that snaked through a patchwork of greens and blues. We crouched behind some rocks for a quick round of bagels and cream cheese. Sam pulled on rain pants and a wool hat, I put my extra pair of socks over my hands, and then we ran along the ridge, completely exposed as we scrambled blindly over slippery rocks.

"We're in the alpine zone!" Sam called back to me as we ran, his voice sounding thin in the pissy wind.

"What?" I yelled.

"Once you get up over forty-five hundred feet, there's only light ground cover and no trees," he yelled back. "These mountains are ancient, and there's not a lot of soil depth. Roots can't take hold of anything. It's a lot like what you'd find in the Arctic Circle!"

"That makes sense," I yelled again. "It's fucking freezing."

"That's why it's good to be prepared," Sam said, turning around to look at me, "because— Oh my god. Where are your rain pants?!"

"I don't have any." My jaw rattled with the *rat-tat-tat* of chattering Muppet teeth. Did Muppets even *have* teeth? It was so cold.

Sam ran over to me. "I thought you wouldn't let me buy you rain pants because you already had some! Are you saying— Oh my god, are these *socks* on your hands? *Cotton socks?* Where are your gloves?"

"It's June!" I said miserably.

"Oh, you poor cutie," he said, rubbing his hands briskly up and down my arms to try to warm them up. Of course it did nothing, but it was nice that he tried. "Oh jeez, your pants are cotton too."

"Is that bad?"

"It's not great," he said. "I'm sorry, I thought everyone knew not to wear cotton for backpacking."

"Why would I know that?"

"I don't know." Sam shrugged, and a ribbon of rain ran down his nose, dripping off the tip. "Everyone knows that."

It took an hour for us to reach the tree line that marked the trail for our descent, and by then my cotton cargo pants and floppy sock mittens were soaked through. After that, it took *another* hour to get to our campsite. I started using my footsteps as a metronome for Disney songs I sang to myself, trying to come up with new lyrics as a distraction from my misery. *No one hikes like Gaston, rides a bike like Gaston, driving west no one takes the Mass Pike like Gaston.*

The campsite was nothing like what I expected or wanted. There were no picnic tables, no fire pits. "No fires allowed," Sam told me when I asked. We had a raised wooden platform for our tent, and a two-minute walk to something called a "compost toilet," which is just a collaboration between the two grossest words in the English language.

"Why don't you have a rest while I set up the tent?" Sam asked, pulling a long, thin nylon bag from his backpack, and from that a few long, thin collapsible metal poles.

"Are you sure? I'm happy to help," I lied, clenching my kneecaps tightly so they didn't pop off and roll away into the den of whatever predator lurked wetly in the shadows, biding its time.

"Yeah, it'll be quick," he said. A few minutes later he told me to go inside the tent and change into my warm pants while he set up the Sterno cans for his camping stove to make dinner.

"I told you," I said, "I don't have any."

"You don't have *rain* pants," Sam said.

"Right," I said, too cold to blush. "I also don't have any *other* pants."

Sam was speechless for a second, probably not with desire. And then he said, "You literally don't have *any other* pants with you?"

"Who needs pants, baby?" I giggled, trying to sound flirty. Even in the midst of what was shaping up to be a crisis, I couldn't help myself from trying to campily sex it up. Ha! Campily. That pun wasn't even on purpose. My brain just does that.

"Come on," Sam said, and steered me into the tent. He stripped off my wet clothes and completely ignored my wiggling in the general direction of his crotch, instead producing his own fleece-lined, waterproof pants and helping me wriggle into them. He zipped the sleeping bags together to make one giant one, tucked me in, then went back outside in the rain for a while. I just lay there shivering. This was not the no-pants party I'd imagined.

He returned with a steaming pot full of rotini and sauce. "Time to play Yum Yum," he said, sliding into the sleeping bag with me.

"Should I take my pants off again?" I asked hopefully.

"Are you kidding?"

" ...Yes?"

He stabbed a few pieces of pasta with a fork and held them toward my mouth. "To warm you from the inside," he said. "I'm treating you for hypothermia. Come on."

I grudgingly took a few bites, but then I hit a wall. "Okay," I said shortly. "I'm done."

"You have to eat," Sam said, stabbing a few more pasta spirals. "Come on. Yum yum."

"Why do you keep *saying* that?"

"It's a game you play when you're backpacking," he said. "You can't have food left over, so when everyone feels full you pass the pot around in a circle and take turns taking bites. Every time you do, you say, 'Yum yum!'"

"What's the point?" I asked, wondering if this was a real thing or if Sam was just messing with me for his own amusement.

"To not have food left over."

"Couldn't we just bring it with us tomorrow?"

Sam looked like I'd asked him why we couldn't just bip bop the deeperdops.

"We don't want to add weight to our packs with leftover cooked pasta," he said. "I mean, I guess I could put it out in the bear box with our other food but—"

"The what?"

"The bear box. A locked box that protects your food from bears. There's one by the outhouse."

"Ohmygod there are seriously bears?!"

"You don't have to worry about bears," he said. "New Hampshire mountain bears like hugs."

"You didn't tell me there would be bears."

"You didn't tell me you weren't bringing pants."

"It was supposed to be a surprise!"

"It is." Sam offered me another bite. "Here we go, *yum yum.*"

I ate all of the damn pasta and cried about maybe dying in the woods. Sam held me all night without a single *I told you so*, and the next morning announced that we should hike out of the woods and check into a hotel, instead of spending the next two days hiking and camping. I cried again, out of sheer relief.

It took five or six hours, but we made it out of the woods, several miles from where we'd left the car. We hitchhiked back to the parking area with a chatty older lady, then drove to a bed-and-breakfast, where the rooms overflowed with wicker chairs and lace curtains and Jesus paraphernalia. I was so happy to be in a nice warm bed with my nice warm Sam that I fell asleep instantly, even under the watchful eye of the son of the deity who made hotels.

We made it home—*Hallelujah! Hooray!*—and I called my parents to fill them in on the whole situation.

"You went camping?" Dad asked, sounding surprised. "Just you and some guy? Alone in a tent?"

"I'm twenty-seven years old, Dad."

"Well," my mother chimed in, "are we going to meet him?"

"Oh, hi, Mom, you're on the line too?"

"I'm on the cordless in the garden," she said. "You should see my clematis this year!"

"The clematis!" Dad echoed proudly.

"You should see Callie," Mom said. Callie was my parents' rescue dog and constant companion. "Whenever I spray the hose she jumps up to drink out of it."

"She gets air!" Dad said.

"Good girl, Cal!" Mom called, and I heard heavy panting in the background. "Jump, Callie! Wheeeeeeee! Hang on, Sar. Callie, wheeeeeee!"

"Do you like this guy?" Dad asked me. "Is it serious?"

"*Dad,*" I groaned. "I don't know."

"It's serious enough to sleep in the woods."

"I guess."

"I like this guy," he said.

"You haven't even met him."

"He got you out of the woods."

"Yeah."

"Even though he shouldn't have taken you into the woods in the first place."

"Your father's idea of roughing it is a hotel without room service." Mom was back. "Callie! Callie, wheeeeeee!"

"Uck, feh," Dad said. "The woods are for bears."

"Sam says New Hampshire bears like hugs," I said.

"Ha!" Dad said. It wasn't a laugh, but a joyful exhalation he always made whenever he was pleased or amazed. It's hard to capture the sound on paper. "I'm telling you, I like this kid."

"We're not kids, Dad."

"You're kids to me, kid," he said.

My father wanted to meet this "kid" who got me out of the woods, so I brought Sam to my parents' house for dinner. Mom grilled the last drops of life out of some steaks, while Sam and Dad chatted over beers. Dad was especially interested in hearing about Sam's plans to apply to business school, since his company worked so closely with universities.

Later, after we'd stuffed ourselves with charred steak and some of my mom's crispy chocolate chip cookies, I slipped out through the garage to the driveway, to call Callie inside so that Mom could give her leftover gristle and lettuce—the dog liked salad with her steak.

Dad followed me out. "You two are going to have very smart children," he said, gesturing inside, where Sam was fielding questions from Mom.

"*Dad!*" I hissed just above a whisper.

"Very smart and very pale," he said.

The very smart and very pale Sam and I stayed together. We moved in together, and, eventually, moved to San Francisco together. We took a few weeks to drive Sam's silver Subaru cross-country, first driving up to Maine to see friends, then back down the East Coast to visit my brother, who was then living in North Carolina. From there we headed west through Tennessee, Missouri, Kansas. Sam wanted to hike and camp his way through the natural beauty of our great land; I wanted to go to Dolly Parton's aptly named Appalachian theme park, Dollywood, and visit weird roadside superlatives like the world's largest chocolate moose. We ended up doing a little bit of both. During the second half of our trip, somewhere between the kitschy Old West–style saloons of Dodge City, Kansas, and the otherworldly canyons of Utah's Zion National Park, Mom called to tell me that my dad had lost his job.

Part II
During

Chapter 8

NICE MOOVES

Unemployment is never fun or fine, even when you're twenty-five and calling it "funemployment" and pretending it's an adventurous opportunity for weekday brunches and finally working on that novel. Which I absolutely did, once.

But Dad was sixty-four and had been with the same company for thirty years. The last time he'd looked for a new job, Jimmy Carter was the president, and lapels were wide enough to land airplanes on.

I guess we could have seen it coming. The country was still clawing its way out of the Great Recession, and everyone was cutting even the teeniest costs. My mom told me that all of my dad's clients decided to do their own marketing and develop virtual programs that "attendees" could complete online.

Dad was outraged.

"This is poppycock!" he yelled at me during a phone call, and I would have laughed at this ridiculous choice of words if he hadn't sounded so upset. "Nobody in their right mind would take an online class if they have the opportunity to go in person. People like experiences! People like materials! There's no way they'll get the same results with sending emails as I do sending beautiful brochures."

"Wait," I said on the phone one night, "you don't use email marketing?! You use mailers? But think of how expensive those are, Dad! Why would anyone spend the money on something that's going to get thrown away most of the time anyway?"

I wish I'd said that more nicely, but it just kind of came out. It was so frustrating to hear Dad frozen in time, to hear him sound so...irrelevant. And old. Your parents aren't supposed to be old; your parents are supposed to be infallible.

Dad didn't say anything. Instead, he hung up on me.

I called back immediately, but my mom answered and told me that Dad had taken the dog for a walk. I could hear him slamming dishes around in the background, though.

"You hurt his feelings, Sar," she said. "He's very sensitive right now."

"I know," I said. "I just want to help him."

"You could help him by being more patient," she said. "He knows he's in trouble here, he just can't admit it yet."

"Can I talk to him?"

"Let him be for now," she said. "He'll call you when he's ready to talk. Right now he's embarrassed. He doesn't want you to think he's old."

"He *is* old," I joked weakly.

I didn't talk to Dad for a week. Finally, he called and asked me to help him navigate his job search. Even though he sounded frustrated, his tone was light, like he'd forgotten that our last conversation ended on an angry note. I guess that wasn't too surprising. The usual MO in our family was to avoid rehashing arguments. It was more comfortable to pretend they'd never happened.

"There's nothing in the paper," he said. "I've been looking every day. Nobody's got any jobs."

"Well," I began slowly, softly, trying not to poke the ole internet bear, "people don't really use the newspaper want ads anymore, Dad. Most companies post job openings online."

"The fakakta internet," he said. "Well, I need you to come over and show me how to do that. Can you come tonight? Bring Sam. Stay for dinner."

"...I moved to San Francisco, Dad."

"Oh. Right."

"Jeez old man, brain fart," I joked.

"Uck, come on. Don't use that word," he said.

I rolled my eyes. Still policing my language, even in my thirties. "Whatever, Dad. Anyway, I can help you the next time I'm home, if that's okay?"

"Sure. Sorry to bother you on this."

"It's no bother, Dad," I said. "I want to help you."

"My daughter, the angel!" he said.

I flew home to Boston, and Sam and I drove out to my parents' house. It's trippy to date someone from your hometown whom you didn't know as a kid. I'd often forget that the back roads and buildings were familiar to him, too, and I found it hard to break an annoying habit I'd inherited from Dad: automatically, absent-mindedly pointing out places with historical significance. Like, *That yellow house was a tavern during the Revolutionary War*, or *That's the river in "Over the River and Through the Wood."*

At dinner, I couldn't help teasing my dinosaur dad about his hang-ups about the internet, and then Sam offered his thoughts on the cost efficiency of online marketing.

Dad didn't like our hot takes on his life. "People want to hold something in their hands!" he cried. "Jesus God, I've been doing marketing for thirty years! The internet is a trend. It's stupid. People want human connection."

————

After dinner, Sam kept my mom company in the kitchen, and I went into a small room that my father had set up as his "office," where he mostly played the classic solitaire game that comes with Windows laptops and bought fake Oriental rugs on eBay. He insisted they were real. Since I could remember—since they'd had an internet connection, probably—my dad had bought $100 rugs off of eBay whenever he felt stressed out. Every room in their house had at least one—even the rooms with wall-to-wall carpeting were doubled up with an Oriental rug or two.

I pulled a kitchen chair up to Dad's desk to peer at his thick brick of a laptop and saw that he'd been looking at a real estate website.

"We're thinking of moving," Dad said. "Someplace smaller. A little cheaper. But we need to stay near Boston because that's where all of my contacts are, and I don't want a long commute to my new job."

This was a surprise. "Oh?" I asked. "You got a new job? You didn't tell me. I thought we were about to look at job listings."

"No," he said. "I mean, when I get a new job. We'll want to move before I start, but I still want to look in the area. Right now my drive's a real beast."

"You mean, it *was*," I corrected.

God. Why do I do that? I've always done that, pounced on tiny inconsistencies and mistakes. I used to think this nasty habit was a compulsive product of insecurity, but I don't know. I think I just like the smug rush of superiority.

"Oh. Right," Dad said.

"Let's start with Monster.com," I said.

Dad hit the home button on his browser—his home page was set to Google.

"Dad," I said impatiently, "you don't need to look up Monster.com; all you need to do is—"

I cut myself off as I watched Dad type "http://www.google.com" into the search bar.

"What are you *doing*?" I asked.

"I needed to look up Monster.com."

"First of all," I said, and pointed to the address bar, "you don't. You can just put 'Monster.com' up in this little box right here. Hell—sorry, heck—you can just put 'Monster,' but *second* of all, Dad. You just used Google to google 'Google.'"

"I did what?" Dad asked, puzzled. I tried to explain a search engine, but I didn't have the language to do it. The internet's been a part of my life for so long, ever since high school when Ace Casey and I would use his family's modem to browse for sex FAQs online. Trying to explain the internet, and search engines, felt a little like trying to explain what the word "and" means, without using it in its own definition.

I just took over the computer and did it for him, and we silently browsed around job sites for a while but didn't see anything.

After a fruitless hour Sam came in from the kitchen and said, "You know, maybe it would be worth it to reach out to some of the places where you'd like to work."

"I want to work at my old job," Dad said.

"...Right," Sam said, tiptoeing as carefully as a peanut vendor in a public school cafeteria, "but that's not an option anymore, right?"

My father huffed a *garrumph*, which sounds like it could be whimsical, but it definitely was not.

"If you want, I'd be happy to help shape up your résumé," Sam said.

"Oh yeah, Dad," I said. "Sam's really good at them."

"I don't have a résumé," Dad said.

"You don't have a *résumé*?" Sam asked.

"I don't like to brag about myself," my father said.

"It's not…*bragging*, Dad," I said. "It's listing work experience, accomplishments, and contributions."

"That's bragging."

It took the rest of dinner, plus a few phone calls from back on the West Coast, to convince my father that a bulleted list of companies, dates, and job descriptions wasn't bragging. Where was that even coming from? I didn't know my dad to be a humble guy. I mean, he wasn't the kind of guy to take out a billboard ad to celebrate his own accomplishments, but he'd always told me to take pride in my work and never sell myself short about it.

Finally, I got an email from him that made me think about this whole thing differently.

It said:

> Thanks for taking the time to look at this
>   It feels a little empty and irrelevant.

He'd attached a Word document that was a perfectly great résumé, listing skills, professional history, education. My eye twitched when I saw "Author," but I was surprised and relieved to see that he'd listed two books about computers:

> *Computing for Profits: 101 of the Best Money-Making Applications for a Personal Computer* (with Allan H. Schmidt, Collier Books, MacMillan Publishing Company)
>   *Marketing Your Software: 26 Steps to Success* (with William G. Nisen and Allan Schmidt, Addison-Wesley Publishing Company)

I called him right away.

"This is a *good* résumé, Dad!" I said. "The jobs should start rolling in."

"I can't find any jobs," he said. "There's nothing in the paper."

"*Dad*." Was I losing my mind? Hadn't we talked about this already? "You're not going to find executive education jobs in the newspaper. You're not going to find *any* jobs that you want to do in the paper. We should look around online to see if we can find openings at companies you'd like to work for."

"How do I do that?"

"I'll help you."

I helped him for the next two years.

That's a heavy sentence, I guess.

My father could not find a job. It was painful for everyone. I don't want to downplay the agony of a two-year job search by summarizing it, but so much of it was tedious, and repetitive. I spent hours researching executive education programs, looking for job listings and contact information, vetting headhunters that might be able to place Dad in a high-level position. I flew back and forth and back and forth between Boston and San Francisco. I sent countless "Hey, check this out!!" emails to Dad; he'd reply with enthusiasm and send me a new version of his résumé. Nothing panned out.

In between the researching and applying and not-panning-outing, I fielded endless requests for computer help from my father, via my mother. "I think the boredom's getting to him," Mom would whisper into the phone when she called with a new iteration of the same question—about how to use the internet, or the printer, or how to access his emails.

I didn't recognize this man who couldn't figure out job searches or his computer. Not just because I'd long idolized my dad as a personal superhero, but because he used to know all of this stuff.

At one point when I was a kid, one of Dad's biggest clients was a major computer company that was an early pioneer in hardware and software. I remember seeing their logo—blocks of letters that looked like typewriter keys—on marketing swag that Dad sometimes brought home. He worked closely with the company's engineers to develop training programs and would have had to develop at least a fundamental understanding of how their products worked.

I don't think Dad loved having a corporate job. But he loved the people he worked with and loved learning new stuff. And Dad was *excited* about computers. He brought one home when I was nine or ten. I think it was a DEC, I can't remember the model. I just remember how cool I thought it was, and how smart my father seemed.

The computer had a green screen and a blinking rectangle cursor, and to boot it up you used a floppy disk the size of a slice of bread. He couldn't wait to show me the command menu, how I could create a new document, or save one to another disk. There was a command to dial up another computer using a telephone line, and when I asked him what that meant, he explained that computers could talk to other computers, to share information. I pictured an anthropomorphic monitor with springy arms, clutching a telephone receiver with one claw and using the other to spin the dial on a rotary, ringing his best pal for a quick chat.

Dad helped me to navigate my first real job search too. When I was in my early twenties and sort of floating aimlessly around Boston, a ghost with nobody to haunt, Dad helped me connect with some old friends and colleagues from his newspaper days.

One kind managing editor took pity on me and gave me a small, fluffy assignment to write some advertorial nonsense. I can't remember. It was probably something they normally assigned to interns. I think they paid me $20. And I was so happy. A real writer, you know? Paid to write. Over time the assignments were more substantial, and eventually I ended up on the writing staff at the very newspaper my dad was working for when he met my mother.

I felt (still feel) like I owed him my career.

So when he'd call to ask me how to check his email, or excitedly announce that he wanted help with an online application for a digital marketing manager position, I dug my nails into my palms and listened. I didn't listen *patiently*, but I did tend to drop whatever I was doing to walk him through checking his email again or submitting his résumé for a job that required digital experience even to just apply for it.

It was just all so sad, to hear and see my father age in real time, and at lightning speed. I thought old men were supposed to wear canvas pants, and take up bird-watching, and join barbershop quartets. Instead, he was stuck in a bittersweet spot, not ready or able to retire, not tech-savvy enough to qualify for or even apply for most of the jobs he was interested in.

While all of this was happening, Sam and I got engaged, and I was trying to plan our wedding.

Wedding planning is a black hole of calligraphic font choices and tunnel vision boards. The details about other people's weddings are insufferable, so I won't bore you with them, except to say that we decided on an ice cream sundae bar instead of cake, and the ice cream place had an option for the staff to dress up as cows. The cow-people were meant for kids' birthday parties but were udderly perfect for the wedding we wanted: one that bucked the traditions of rubber chicken on fancy plates and bridesmaids smothered in taffeta. That word always makes me think of *Young Frankenstein*, when Gene Wilder tries to passionately clutch Madeline Kahn and she flinches, because she doesn't want to crush her dress. *Taffeta, darling*, she says, and Gene replies, *Taffeta, sweetheart*.

No, she says. *The dress is taffeta! It wrinkles so easily.*

Dad called for computer help one day as I was in the thick of an online wedding dress search.

"Taffeta, darling," he said.

"Taffeta, sweetheart," I said distractedly as I scrolled through a website dedicated to unconventional weddings. Unconventional brides are no less insufferable than traditional ones as it turns out, only instead of nitpicking floral arrangements, they're putting fireflies in jars and offending their conservative relatives with vegan meals and home-brewed beer. I have a friend who went to a hippie wedding where the couple fermented their own champagne. Everyone who drank it ended up hallucinating. *That's* a party.

"Is this a bad time?" Dad asked. "Sorry to bother you again, but my laptop stopped working so I can't get my emails."

"Just log on from Mom's computer, Dad."

"I can't get my emails on her computer; they're *my* emails."

I closed my eyes and thought of the English lavender I was considering for boutonnieres.

"You said your laptop isn't working?" I asked through my teeth. Were we really going to have this conversation again? "What's going on this time?"

"I keep hitting buttons but nothing's happening."

"You need to be *specific*, Dad," I said, so irritated by this infinite loop of email bullshit. I was trying so hard to be a good and grateful daughter. I was also trying so hard to find the perfect peacock feather fascinator. I suppose those things don't have to be mutually exclusive, but in that particular moment it was truly one or the other. "Is the screen frozen?" I prompted. "Is it blank? Are you just having trouble using Google again?"

"The screen is totally black," he said, sounding just as raw as my own nerves felt. "I keep pressing buttons, but, nothing."

"Is the computer...on?" I asked.

"I have no idea if the goddamned computer is on!" he cried. "How do I turn it on?"

"...Are you serious?"

"Yes, I'm serious!"

"Don't be mad at me, Dad!"

"I'm not mad at you, I'm mad at the computer."

"Just use Mom's," I said, and he roared an unwritable noise of ire.

"I can't get my emails on Mom's!" he yelled.

These recursive conversations about emails reminded me of standing in front of a mirror and looking into another mirror, or the inside of a prism, or the cover of a prog rock album.

"The computer just stresses you out, Dad," I said. "Why don't you take a break from it for a few days? I'll do some more job searching on my end and then call you if I find anything."

"You can hold off on the job search. I'm starting a business. Writing more books."

I froze.

Did he mean *the* books? Were we really about to do this, to come clean about how, ha ha, my father wrote sex books and, ha ha, I've always known? What would that mean for our relationship? Would it mean anything at all? Would it just be a dreaded difficult conversation to bumble through, or turn into an existential exploration of my father's purpose, or my own? Fuck, the suspense was killing me. The suspense was—

Oh. The suspense was my fault. It was my turn to talk.

"Um...," I said, puncturing that can of worms so very cautiously, "*more* books, Dad?"

"Yeah," Dad said, like it was nothing, like we'd been talking about his books for years.

"Like...computer books? Or..."

I braced myself for an extremely unprecedented, extremely difficult conversation. But instead, Dad said he was inspired by his and Mom's obsession with their hose-drinking rescue pup, Callie. He wanted to create a whole line of books, T-shirts, and "canine lifestyle" products under the name Dog Child, and he had already reconnected with his old illustrator and creative partner, Marty Riskin.

Marty did all of the illustrations for the sex books and is also a political cartoonist and fine art painter. I met him a bunch of times when I was a little girl. Dad always described him as "my artist friend." When I was in the third grade, Marty illustrated a story that I wrote about my classroom pet, a white rat named Whiskers: "Whiskers Takes Karate Lessons." He and Dad turned it into a large-format paperback book, and I still have it. It's one of my most prized possessions.

Even so, when I think of Marty I think of buxom cartoon women, and that orange cat with heavy bedroom eyes. So a "canine lifestyle" book was a huge relief.

Dad said he'd found an investor for the books who would cover all of the production costs, and that he'd booked himself a booth at a trade show for the "gift" industry. Not bad for a man who couldn't turn his computer on. A few weeks later, he sent me an email with a finished manuscript for "Dog Child:

The Big Dog Book," and it was really cute! A sincere ode to pets that was full of dopey Dad jokes and joyful pen-and-ink sketches. The table of contents seemed pretty direct too. What a relief.

Dad was really excited about his new business venture, and Mom was too. Every time I talked to one of them, they mentioned "the family business," and I thought maybe that meant that my mother was in on it, too, until Dad told me that he meant this business to be my "inheritance." He wanted to leave it to me when he died.

"I don't want to talk about you *dying*, Dad, come on," I said. Everyone I knew was so far away from dying. These days people live until they're in their nineties. Dad was only in his sixties. There were many road-trip word games and irritating conversations about emails in our future.

Dad, Marty, and their investor decided to officially start their own publishing imprint, Impish Publishing, so they could create all kinds of new works. Dad wanted to write a daily blog on their website, so I set one up and made him a step-by-step user's guide for it. But ole Can't Get My Emails Alterman couldn't figure out how to use the blog, even with my guidance, so I suggested he just email me the text and I would post the blogs for him.

Big mistake.

Big, world-rocking, mind-fucking mistake.

It was fine at first. He sent me some tongue-in-cheek copy for his bio, and an inaugural blog post that featured a few silly cartoons from their "Library of Funny."

And then, on July 13, 2011, my father asked me to post this:

Sex After 40

In the end, it's all about sex. But don't take our word for it.

In his book, *Programming the Universe*, MIT professor Seth Lloyd calls the invention of sex a great revolution "dwarfing all that followed...a tour de force," and pays it the ultimate MIT compliment: "Sex is not only fun, it is good engineering practice."

Then he goes on to explain the universe, blah, blah, blah. And we're kicking ourselves for not getting a degree in engineering. Who knew?

The best we can do at this point is become a sex missionary, spreading the word and doing good sex deeds. So we're writing a book of our own: "Sex After 40."

You probably want to see a few excerpts:

Introduction

While sex in your 20s and 30s is a hundred yard dash, sex in your 40s is a languid, passionate trip through a garden of lush eroticism, sensual interpersonal connection, and steamy, kinky verbal and physical exchanges.

You wish.

More likely, your rakish good looks are heading south, your scented massage oils have gone sour, and it has been a long time since you've had any.

Which can happen frequently to people who are over 40.

Which is why you need this book.

Rediscovering Foreplay

Woody Allen said that sex is like playing bridge. If you don't have a good partner, you need a good hand.

What makes a good partner? It's you, paying attention to the little things that will put your partner in the mood: An unexpected compliment; a surprise, lingering kiss on the nape of the neck; sexy, romantic wordplay; a discreet, intimate caress in a public place; leaning over and planting a wet one on your partner's lap at a red light; an outrageous, whispered promise of sexual performance that would require a safety net and a dozen circus roustabouts to fulfill, and so on.

> We call this "foreplay." It is a substitute for ripping off all
> the buttons, unhooking all the clasps, untying all the knots,
> and unzipping all the zippers that are keeping you from
> getting laid.

Dad attached two other files to that email: a pen-and-ink
illustration of a naked man humping the number 40; and another
called "The Sex Missionary," which showed a balding man, in
monk's clothing, tossing handfuls of condoms into the sky.

There was no explanation for any of this, no comment, no
"Hey, sorry if this is weird, but…" It was just a casual email from
Dad to daughter, a casual condom monk, casual sex.

"Speechless" doesn't really cover how this email left me.

Another person might laugh at their dad's dirty-old-man she-
nanigans. Hell (damn!), my dad had been a dirty old man since
before I was born, and I'd known it, and kept that knowledge a
secret. That's kind of the point. None of this is sinister, or sala-
cious. My father wrote some corny porn/porny corn that brought
joy to the world and, as far as I could tell, caused no pain for
anyone but me. But until hitting send on this 345-word email,
he'd never said anything even remotely sexual in my presence,
or even in my direction. Over decades of compartmentalizing
his life into a bento box of personas, my father had never once
dropped the Dad act with me.

This email felt off.

Maybe he sent this to me by accident, I thought. *Maybe I'm
overreacting.*

I decided that he must have sent me the blog post and monk
humps by accident, so I said nothing to him, or anyone. Mom
would have been mortified. Sam would have laughed. I didn't
feel like dealing with either of those reactions.

But then, a few days later, Dad sent me this:

7/19/2011

Orgasms After 40: How to Make Them Better and More Frequent

[The second in a series of excerpts from our forthcoming book, "Sex After 40"]

Experts agree that people over 40 basically experience three kinds of orgasms:

1. The Dead Man's Last Hurrah, where one partner struggles for fulfillment while pinned under the dead weight of the other, who has fallen asleep in mid lunge. Two problems here. First, this is inexcusable. Second, it could have a devastating impact on alimony payments sometime in the future.
2. Runners Take Your Mark. The most common orgasm among struggling 40s, it occurs from 3 to 11 seconds after the start of intercourse. Nonetheless, frazzled 40s are happy to have the 11 seconds all to themselves.
3. A Night at the Opera is an orgasm that could be set to music. Nothing short of a passion play, it is accompanied by high-pitched, reedy wailing, an excess of emotion, and deep, penetrating sobs of gratitude. The woman person is also happy. This one is the gold standard.

It is not a surprise that many people over 40 are either dissatisfied with the quality of their orgasms and want to make them better, or with the quantity of their orgasms and

want to have more of them. Like learning to play the bag-
pipes, this is a matter of practice, alone in a room, where
no one can hear you.

The woman person.
Deep, penetrating sobs of gratitude.
Our forthcoming book, "Sex After 40."

I had to call my father. I didn't want to. But I had to know
what was going on with him.

"Hi, Dad," I said when he answered my call, "I'm just going
to jump in, okay? You sent me a post, and—"

"Whadja think?" he asked, his mouth full of something that
crunched like jumbo corn nuts, or like somebody else's teeth.

"What are you eating?"

Crunch crunch munch. "Turdur juhs uhs."

"What?"

Munch munch crunch. "Turdur juhs uhs."

"Okay, Dad. This is serious, so if you need to finish eating, I'll
call you back."

He made a noise of protest. "Wait!" he said. *Chomp. Gulp.*
"Trader Joe's O's. Mom gets them for me. It's like chewing on a
bowl of stale goose poopies. Just god-awful."

"Then why do you eat them?"

"I don't know," Dad said limply. "They're there."

He sounded so small, and so sad, filling his mouth with cereal
he hated, just to have something to do. That might be the saddest
thing I've ever heard. It softened me.

"I got your post," I said. "And, um, I'll put it up today, okay?"

"That's great, honey!" he said, then took a huge, satisfied bite.
Crunch crunch munch.

Three months later, in October 2011, Sam and I got married

under a moon-shaped skylight in a midcentury modern non-denominational chapel in Cambridge, Massachusetts. It was almost perfect. We wrote our own vows. Daniel's wife, Jesse, made my bouquet. I forgot to wear a bra.

Mom and Dad both walked me down the aisle, the slowest and fastest walk of my life. I just looked at Sam, standing at the foot of a white marble altar, freshly shaven and probably just as hungover as I was from the post–rehearsal dinner rager we staged at a nearby Irish bar, like utter bozos.

When we reached the head of the aisle, and it was time to hand me off to Sam, Mom hugged me, then hugged Sam, then took her seat. Dad shook Sam's hand, then gave me a peck on the cheek and squeezed my hand. He looked so happy.

"Love you, Dad," I whispered. Then I took a step toward Sam, and felt my strapless dress slip dangerously down my unswathed cleavage. Shit. My dad was standing on the train of my dress.

"You're standing on me," I whispered to him. He didn't understand what I was saying, so I whispered again. He just smiled the same happy smile, which now looked blank to me. "Dad," I hissed, louder. "You're *standing* on me." But my father was frozen—bewildered, possibly, by standing front and center before nearly two hundred guests.

I had no idea what to do. I'm not really ruffled by standing in front of a large crowd, but I was worried that maybe Dad was thrown off by his own nerves. I didn't want to embarrass him, but I also didn't have a next move.

Finally, Sam stepped forward and touched Dad's elbow, then gently directed him toward his seat in the front row, next to my mom.

I meant to ask my father about the dress-step, and to laugh

about it with him, but I couldn't find him after the ceremony, and then at the reception everyone was distracted by the ice cream cows. One of them could breakdance.

Nice mooves, I thought, and, wherever he was, I knew my dad was thinking it too.

Chapter 9

GLUG GLUG GLUG

Oriental rugs are heavier than you might think. You might not have thought about it at all, actually—I certainly hadn't, until I had to fireman-carry thirty-two of them by myself, one by one, up two flights of stairs.

The winter after my wedding, in early 2012, Mom and Dad sold their house and moved to a rental up on the North Shore, in an old mill town just across the river from a historic fishing village turned prosperous seaport turned fancy seaside vacation destination, where tourists come for chowdah and locals own boats with names like *Seas the Day*, and *Naut On My Watch*, and *Dock Lobstah*.

There's a maritime museum in an old customshouse on the main street, and it reminded me of a squat, stone toad that Mom kept on the windowsill above her kitchen sink. I flew home to help them move in.

To get to the North Shore from Boston's Logan Airport, you have to take a subway to the station beneath what used to be the Boston Garden, before it was torn down and rebuilt and renamed for a series of corporate sponsor overlords. Then you squeeze your way through commuters during rush hour, or tourists during leaf-peeping season, or students during orientation week, or Celtics fans during basketball season, or Bruins fans during hockey season, or Red Sox fans year-round, because Sox fandom knows no season.

From there you grab a commuter train north, and spend an hour rumbling along from Boston to other, smaller cities, then along lush marshlands and the peaceful fields and forests of the suburbs. The train station is near the mouth of a river that spills into the sea. It's quaintly, New Englandly beautiful there.

So moving day came, and I took a plane to the subway to the train up to the North Shore. It was snowing, but when I arrived, Dad was waiting for me on the outdoor platform, hands shoved into the pockets of his cracked brown leather bomber jacket. He smiled widely when he saw me, and laughed his signature little *ha*, and it floated on a cloud of frozen breath. He'd changed since the last time I saw him. His beard was more salt than pepper, his curly hair fluffy and thinning.

"Dad!" I smiled too. "You could have stayed in the car. It's so cold."

He gave me a huge hug and kiss and took the handle of my rolling suitcase. "I always come get you," he said.

"I know, but, it's *cold*. You look cold."

"You look good," he said as we arrived at his SUV, parked across three spaces.

"Thanks. You look old," I teased, and immediately regretted it as I watched him fumble with the car keys. First he couldn't get them out of his pocket, then he pressed the alarm button instead of unlock. He shut it off, then struggled to hoist my suitcase into the trunk.

"I'm just kidding, Dad," I said, though not quickly enough. "You look great."

"I feel great."

"That's great."

We climbed into the car, and when Dad turned the keys in the ignition the heat blasted like a hellfire, and "The Girl from Ipanema" thundered from the speakers. It's one of Dad's favorite songs. It's supposed to be sweet and soft.

"Should we do some job stuff while we're— Jesus, Dad!"

After my father zipped out of the parking lot, he'd suddenly cut a right turn so closely that the car rumbled into a curb.

"Almost missed the goddamned turn," he said. "Sorry, honey, the sun's in my eyes."

We drove straight to the new place, and I moved a staggering amount of rugs from their beast of a rental truck into the house. Mom said they'd given ten or fifteen rugs away before the move, and that Dad had been buying them compulsively. "It calms him down," she said when he wasn't listening. "And they're great rugs. We got good deals. They're 100 percent authentic. Good price."

She told me that the move had scared Dad back into job searching, that Dog Child had proven to be less of an empire and more of an exercise in dipping his toes back into publishing. I wondered if she knew about "Sex After 40." Of course I didn't ask.

———

Instead, I made my father a LinkedIn profile.

When I called to ask him for a few lines about his work history, I explained what I was doing.

"It's a social media site," I said, "for professional networking."

"I don't use social media. I'm not a teenager."

"I know, but that's not what this is. LinkedIn is for connecting with people you've worked with—"

"I can just call them."

"—and with people who work for companies you're interested in."

"I'm not interested in companies, I'm interested in people."

"... Okay."

"I just want to work. I don't care who I work for."

"... Okay."

"Okay."

I tried to create a LinkedIn profile anyway, but when I entered his email address, it said that an account with that address already existed. So I looked, and, yes, Dad already had a LinkedIn page. It didn't have a lot of information on it, or a photo, so I called to ask about it.

"Oh yeah," he said. "LinkedIn. I have that."

"... Okay, old man," I said, trying to sound breezy. "Well, your profile could use some work. You have, like, zero work history—"

"That's bragging."

"—and there's no photo. Can you send me one?"

"How do I do that?" he said, and I told him to have Mom help. He emailed me a link to an image of the Israeli rabbi Chaim Kanievsky. I think it was supposed to be a joke.

Sam walked into the kitchen as I was hunched over like a cartoon witch, free-falling down a rabbit hole of profile updates and job listings.

"Baby," he said, "your poor back. Doesn't it hurt to sit like that?"

"Mmm-hmm," I said absentmindedly, peering at a post from an executive education program in Pennsylvania. "I found a job near where Dad grew up; maybe he'd be willing to move."

Sam sat down across from me, at our little white table in our little yellow breakfast nook. It was my favorite part of our San Francisco apartment, besides the tiny pond in our backyard. Nobody gets a backyard in San Francisco, much less a tiny pond, much *less* discovers, after several years of thinking the pond was empty, that a few goliath goldfish are alive at the bottom, surviving off of bugs. Possibly other fish.

"I think this is unhealthy," he said. "You're obsessing over your father's job search. I don't like what it's doing to you."

"He needs my help," I said.

"It would probably help him more if you let him manage his own job search."

"He can't," I snapped. "He doesn't understand how to reach out to people at companies he wants to work for."

"Don't you think that if your dad can't understand computers then maybe it's time for him to take himself out of the job market?" Sam asked. "It would be different if he weren't trying to get an executive-level office job. But I can't imagine that he'd get hired at the kind of company he wants to work for, in the kind of role he wants to have, without having basic computer skills."

Sam was trying to be gentle, I know. But I was feeling so sensitive and sad about my hopelessly unemployed and unemployable father that I could have divorced, killed, and eaten him, in no particular order. I just wanted my dad to find a job, so we could all stop feeling like my parents' future was a giant question mark.

"It would be good," he continued, "if we could start focusing on our own family, you know?"

Shit. I knew where this was going. Sam wanted kids. I...did...not? He brought it up a lot. I...did...not.

"I know you're ready to have kids, babe—" I started.

"I thought you were too?"

"Why do you think that?" I said, annoyed. "I'm still figuring out my career, I need to figure out what's going on with my parents. I don't want to ruin my body; we'll never have a life again."

"You have a lot of excuses," Sam said, and I think he was trying to tease me but it pissed me off.

"They're not *excuses*, they're *reasons*."

"I know," he said. "I was teasing. We used to banter more, it was fun."

"Life doesn't feel fun right now," I said.

"Don't you think it would be fun to have a little baby?" Sam asked. "I can't wait!"

I could.

My parents had never pressured me to give them grand-children, or even asked if it was a possibility. I know a ton of people who've endured those kinds of boundary violations for years, and I think it's gross. To be honest, I thought kids were gross in general. I knew, and know, a lot of people who became parents and instantly became different people. The last thing I wanted was to disappear into a diaper pail, or a roster of class-room moms, or a suburb like the one that made young me feel like an unlovable loser.

Although Sam and I were going nowhere with our baby arguments, Dad, at least, had seen some progress.

"Do you know what LinkedIn is?" he asked on the phone one day. His calls had increased from a few times a week to a few times a day. Sam started leaving the room whenever my parents' number popped up on my caller ID.

"Dad…," I said. "You're fucking with me, right?"

"Watch that language," he said. "LinkedIn, it's a connecting thing, for job people."

Was he trolling me? "I *know*," I said. "We just talked about your LinkedIn profile a few weeks ago."

"Anyway," Dad said, "a guy I did some work with at Harvard, nice guy, he wrote me an endorsement. This guy's a big deal. I think I'm getting a job."

Then my mother jumped on the phone too.

"This guy's a big deal," she echoed. "He knows your father's the best in the business."

"Guys," I said, "this doesn't mean anything. People write endorsements on LinkedIn all the time."

"The best in the business," Mom said again. "Everyone knows that. Dad's getting a job offer any second."

What reality are you living in? I thought. *Is it nice there?*

"What did this endorsement say?" I asked through my teeth. Here I was going to say something about how tightly my teeth were clenched, and maybe make a butthole joke, but I ultimately passed. It's not that I'm above butthole jokes, just that I think all of the good ones have already been written.

"'Ira is a creative genius,'" Mom trilled. "'I would recommend him for just about anything he wants to do.'"

"And I thought, 'I'll be damned,'" Dad said. "I knew he liked my work, but that's a hell of a compliment. A creative genius. I should call him to say thank you."

"You don't need to do that, Dad."

"Sara's right," Mom added. "Just wait for him to call you about the job and you can thank him then."

"Hang on," I said. "'*The* job?' Is there an actual job?"

"Sounds like there's going to be!" Mom said.

"'A creative genius,'" Dad said again. "'I'll be damned."

"*Guys*," I said. "This is just how LinkedIn *works*. Someone writes something nice about you, then you're supposed to write something nice about them."

"He said I'm a creative genius." Dad was like a dog clutching a bone. Or its butthole. There it is.

"It's just like for vanity," I said. "You're collecting little compliments. Then, when you apply for an *actual* job—"

"Oh, there *will* be a job," Mom said.

"—you can include a link to your LinkedIn profile, and whoever's hiring can see that so-and-so person from such-and-such company said something nice about you."

"He said I'm—" Dad began.

"A creative genius, I *know*," I snapped, pulling out my laptop and pulling up Dad's profile, to see this for myself. There it was, writ large. Some guy thought my father was a creative genius and had posted to that effect... three years ago.

"Dad," I said, "this endorsement is from 2010."

"So?"

"It's 2013."

"So?"

"So... don't you think that if he were going to call and offer you a job, he would have done it? It's been three years."

"Oh," he said, and it was clear how disappointing this reality was. "Well, it's okay, because I picked up a little copywriting with one of my old seminars."

"That's great, Dad! Tell me about it."

"Brochure copy for MIT. And I have an idea for a new program about the psychology of leadership."

"Nobody's ever done anything like it," my mother added.

"I'm going to tell them about it when I hand in this copy," Dad said. "Hey, want to see a house we're thinking about?"

"A house?" I asked. "Thinking about for what?"

"Well, we're not staying in a rental forever," Mom said. "Now that Dad's got work again, we're going to buy something. Small," she added. "But with enough space for you when you come to visit."

"A *house*," Sam echoed when I told him. "Your parents are buying a *house*? They have no income!"

"My dad got some freelance work!" I argued. "And it could lead to a job."

"You sound like your mom," Sam teased.

"Fuck you!" I snapped.

"Come on, baby," he said. "You think freelance copywriting is a reliable or lucrative enough source of income for your parents to buy a house?"

"They get Social Security!" I said, but he was right.

"They should keep renting," Sam continued. "It makes the most financial sense. I don't understand why they'd want to move again, they *just moved*."

"It just feels like that to you because when you were a kid you never moved," I said. "This is just what they do."

It's true. When I was growing up we were constantly in a state of trying to sell our house to buy another. I spent a lot of weekends at a lot of open houses, scampering through other people's homes with my brother and arguing about which one of us would get the bigger bedroom. We didn't actually move that much, just from the house I was born in, to the house where we lived until I was eight, to the house where we lived until I was fifteen, to the house where we lived until I went to college, to my parents' house near Henry Ford's gristmill, to the North Shore rental.

Maybe that *is* a lot.

"Well," he said, "I just think they're in a terrible position to buy a house."

"You always say that renting is like throwing money in the garbage!" I yelled.

"I wouldn't say that," he said. "Sometimes it makes more sense to rent, like when you're on a low fixed income. It's less risky."

I didn't answer, just stormed outside to drink most of a bottle of wine myself, by the miraculous fish pond.

The next day, while Sam was at work, I shot him an instant message.

me: I'm sorry. I'm just sad about my parents

me: I want to fix their problems, and I know I can't

Sam: You don't need to fix their problems, you just need to be a good daughter

me: I think I'm finally doing that

me: so that's good

But then…

me: I made the mistake of calling my mother

me: They have decided that they can not afford to buy a house, so they're looking at rentals in north carolina.

me: Also my dad has his head stuck halfway in the oven because it just hit him that he's not going to get a job

me: PASS THE ZOLOFT

Sam: glug glug glug glug

Sam: (assuming you can get zoloft in liquid form)

me: No that's the wine i'll use to wash it down

Sam: Terrific!

me: UGH

me: ugh ugh ugh

me: I do not know what to do

Sam: Their plans change multiple times a week, I think it helps to take the long view

me: I can't take the long view because i don't know what reasonable parameters are

me: Like, I don't know how much money they actually have, etc.

Sam: I just mean try not to be buffeted around by daily proclamations

me: UGH

Sam: Parents do the darndest things!

me: haha

me: It's not that I'm worried about where they will live, I'm worried that they're sad and defeated all the time, and I'm worried that their relationship is suffering

Sam: If you keep worrying like this it will probably fray your last remaining nerves

me: GLUG GLUG GLUG

And then...

me: OK AFTER ANNOUNCING TEARFULLY YES-TERDAY THAT SHE THOUGHT THAT BUYING A HOUSE WAS A TERRIBLE IDEA, MOM JUST CALLED TO TELL ME THAT THEY ARE NOW GOING TO PUT AN OFFER ON A CONDO

me: ALL CAPS

Sam: OH I SEE ALL CAPS

Sam: but that's great they found something they like!

me: is it?

me: IS IT?

me: because yesterday they "didn't have enough money in the bank to sustain buying a house without finding another source of income"

me: and now they want to buy a house

Sam: I think if you demand consistency from your parents you're going to completely go insane

He was right, of course. And of course, my parents didn't get the condo they put in an offer on. Mom called me in a panic about it, and I flew home to go look at more-affordable houses with them. It was pretty brutal. We met up with a faux-optimistic broker who took us to a few homes in my parents' price range, and they were all basically falling apart.

Mom cried silently about it on the drive home, and Dad reached over to gently rub her arm.

"It's okay, honey," he said. "We'll be able to afford something better once I have a job." Then he drifted into the traffic lane next to us, and a car swerved out of our SUV's way. The driver punched the horn and gave us all possible fingers.

"Careful, Dad!" I cried. Mom didn't say anything.

My phone buzzed. It was a perfectly timed text from my old friend Marc, and it read:

> Wanna join me for an incredibly sad Austrian film about an elderly French woman dying?

I did. Given the fragile state I was in—watching from the backseat while my parents came undone—I shouldn't have, but I did.

Said sad Austrian film was *Amour*.

"There is a great deal that is difficult to watch here," wrote *New York Times* film critic Manohla Dargis, "the indignities of a debilitating illness included, and the equally harsh pain of witnessing a great love, a longtime companion, slowly fade away."

Marc's a music critic and pop culture writer, and he's one of the kindest people I know. Also, a big butthead.

I don't really mean that. That's just a thing we do—for most of our fifteen-year friendship we've pretended to hate each other. If he were looking over my shoulder right now, he'd snort and say, *Pretending*, while making finger quotes. And then, seeing what I've typed, he'd say, *They're called AIR QUOTES, Sara.* And then I'd tell him what a big dumb butthead he is.

Anyway, every year, for fun, he goes to see all of the Best Picture nominees before the Oscars. He calls it a pilgrimage. I call it going to the movies. Either way, Marc's a pretty good person to sit next to while witnessing indignity on the big screen.

I mostly prefer to see movies alone. It started in high school, when I drove myself one lonely, stormy, post–Ace Casey breakup Saturday night to see *The Craft*, a cultish cautionary tale of unbridled teen girl vengeance wherein a coven of miniskirted misfits use witchcraft to harness the power of the universe and, like, hex shit. I loved sitting by myself in the dark, with nobody to put their sticky hands all over my Twizzlers, or tease me about covering my eyes during suspenseful parts. I hate suspense. I hate not knowing how something is going to end. Or suspecting, but having to wait awhile for confirmation.

I didn't know anything about *Amour*, and I welcomed the distraction with overstretched arms, writing back to Marc: *Where? When?* We made plans to meet up in Kendall Square, Cambridge, to torture ourselves and each other.

If you missed *Amour*, as I now wish I had, it's the wrist-slitting story of Anne, an elderly and sophisticated retired music teacher played by Emmanuelle Riva, who has a stroke in her kitchen. Her husband, Georges (Jean-Louis Trintignant), an equally elderly and equally retired music teacher, spends the rest of the film caring for Anne as she transforms into an incontinent stranger. While Anne can still speak coherently, she makes Georges promise that he'll never put her in a nursing home, and he stays true to his word, even as the strain of daily spoon-feeding and adult diaper changing makes him resentful and impatient.

Eventually, he smothers her.

It's a mercy killing, for mutual mercy. Georges and Anne are relieved of their personal agonies, and it brings them peace. This is all just a clunky summary. I majored in film studies and should be ashamed of myself. Sorry, college.

After Georges kills his wife, he surrounds her body with flowers, seals the bedroom door, traps a pigeon in a blanket, cradles it lovingly, and sets it free. During that tender pigeon scene, Marc made a strange noise. I turned to make fun of him for being such a sappy loser and found that he was staring at me, concerned. Confused? His dumb face is hard to read.

Anyway, then I realized that *my* dumb face was weeping every liquid a face is capable of weeping; we're talking openly, silently dripping, snotting, sweating, drooling. I lifted a sleeve to my cheek and could tell, based on pure volume, that I'd been doing all of these things for a while.

"Are you okay?" he whispered.

I wasn't.

"My dad...something...is wrong," I choked out, and the people in front of me did that exasperated twist-around you do to seat-kicking children on flights. "He's just...so...different and...distracted and...I'm so worried and...I think something's really wrong and...they're not telling me..."

Marc didn't say anything, just handed me the handkerchief he keeps in his pocket for what he calls "Southern gentlemanly occasions." I like to picture the handkerchief tenderly mopping a sweaty forehead or signaling an unconditional surrender.

I cried for the rest of the movie and kept it up through the credits. I didn't have anything specific to cry about, beyond over-whelming pity and fear and love for an aging man who seemed to be losing his way.

When the lights came on I was too embarrassed to look at Marc, and he was either too embarrassed or kind, I GUESS, to say anything about my face or its general sop, so we just left.

Outside the theater, a pigeon promptly swooped in and landed at my feet. It was, how you say, *cinématique*, and I burst into fresh tears, gave Marc a quick hug, then sprinted off to find a burrito to eat on the train back through the city and the marshland, back up to my parents, to the sea.

———

I showed Marc what I wrote about when we went to the movies, to make sure we remembered it the same way, and he said, "I'd add a coda wherein I point out that *Amour* did not, in fact, win Best Picture. But that's me."

———

Somehow, somehow, in 2013, my parents managed to buy a condo in a neighboring town that my mother disdainfully de-scribed as "a real honky-tonk kind of place, but it's all we can afford." I'm not sure what she meant by that, but there *was* a nearby establishment called Kitten's Gentlemen's Club, which had weekly drag nights and "shower shows," and a bar that had free comedy and cornhole nights. Not the same night.

I flew home to move rugs again.

The honky-tonk condo community was a few minutes' drive

to the beach and a few minutes' walk to a farm that sold native plants and hosted local craft bazaars. Mom took me to check it out. My favorite vendor was a woman who specialized in restoring, or perhaps exorcising, vintage porcelain baby dolls. Then she soldered their freshly painted heads and limbs to antique coffee cans. As we walked home, and as I regretted not snapping up one of those Frankenbabies, Mom told me they planned to stay in the honky-tonk condo until my dad found full-time work, which she insisted would definitely be soon. By then he'd been out of work for four years.

"Then we'll move closer to Boston," she said. "That's where all of the jobs are."

When my visit was over, as Dad was driving me to the train station so I could do the public transit slog all over again, we passed by the comedy and cornhole place. He said that a cornhole sounded like something you'd want to protect if you were in prison.

Then he said solemnly, "I wanted to talk to you about something. I'm getting the business going again."

"Dog Child?" I asked.

"Another book," he said. "One that I was working on a few years ago, but it could use your touch. It was inspired by your wedding."

"That's so sweet, Dad!" I said. "What's it called?"

"'The Naughty Bride,'" my father said. "'An Indecent Wedding Night Guide.' So virgins understand how to please their men. It'll be great for bachelorette parties."

Oh my god.

I thought we were done with this? I thought the sex books had maybe been a passing fad? Or a fever dream? He hadn't mentioned sex to me in so long, it was such a relief. And now, out of nowhere, Dad's sex-writing aspirations rear their ugly head? Come *on*, there has to be a better way to say that so it doesn't sound like a dick joke.

"…I'm…sorry?" I asked.

"I actually already wrote it," he said. "But it could use a refresh. A woman's touch."

Dad said he thought "bachelorettes" would go insane for "The Naughty Bride," either as a gag gift (and he chuckled at the double entendre of "gag") or as a legitimate and approachable how-to for nervous women. I considered throwing myself from his car the next time he slowed down for a light. He wasn't driving that fast. Shit, no, all of my stuff was in the trunk. I at least needed my wallet, to get back on the plane and get the h-e-double hockey sticks out of this shit show.

I should have said something earlier, back when he sent me that "Sex After 40" blog post. I could have stopped this. Fuck. I could stop it now. We were alone in a car, this would be a spectacular opportunity to force my dad to finally fess up to *Games You Can Play with Your Pussy*, and explain himself. But instead, I just said: "No."

"Oh," Dad said, looking taken aback. "I just thought, you know, you're a writer, and your old man could really use some help."

"Sorry, Dad," I said. "I, um, don't have a lot of time right now."

"Oh," he said, disappointed. We arrived at the train station in silence, and Dad hopped out to take my suitcase out of the trunk and to give me one last kiss on the cheek, with an exaggerated *mwah!*

"Bye, Dad," I said, rubbing my cheek where his beard had scratched me. It was getting long.

"Good-bye, sweetie," he said. "If you change your mind about the book, let me know, okay? I know you'd make it better."

I kissed him back on his papery forehead. "Okay, Dad."

There were no ticket machines or booths at this station; you could only buy tickets on board, for cash. I'd forgotten to get another ticket, forgotten to get cash. My change purse was no help—it was packed with nickels and foil-wrapped wads of old gum. The fare collector stopped by my seat and found me elbows-deep in my suitcase, rooting around for change underneath a pile of dirty underpants, and crying about the old, weird man my father was becoming, or had become. The collector waived the fare, gave me a pat on the shoulder, and handed me a tissue. I bet he'd seen it all, or, at least, seen a lot.

Chapter 10

FAMILY BUSINESS

"I want this to be the year of the baby," Sam announced to me one night over plastic take-out containers of mediocre Chinese dumplings.

"I thought this was the year of the horse," I joked, gesturing toward the paper Chinese zodiac place mats that had come with our order. Sam said nothing.

Read the room, I thought, spearing a floppy shumai and bracing myself for another argument about children, and whether or not we should have them.

I pushed Sam for babies early in our relationship. We were twenty-seven when we met, and I was approaching thirty with the silent anxiety of any woman who'd internalized a lifetime of perceived inadequacies. Thirty. I thought that by thirty, I was supposed to be married, and have kids, and generally have my shit together. That's what the lives of my most successful friends looked like.

For Sam, love unfolds mathematically. A couple dates for X number of years, then gets engaged for Y number of months, marries once, and has Z^1 number of children, wherein $Z = 2$. He refused to hurry things along just because the magic and realism of age thirty made me feel hysterical.

At some point, I don't know, we switched. By the time Sam finally felt the tickety-tock of his reproductive clock, I'd already turned thirty, then thirty-one, thirty-two, thirty-three. I had crinkles around my eyes and red in my checking account. I had vast holes in my résumé from the times I'd tried to launch a freelance writing career, which mostly meant splitting my days between grinding out clickbait headlines and thin articles for a digital marketing company, and grinding through midmorning TRX classes.

I knew Sam would be a great dad. I could picture him enthusiastically building LEGO castles, and swinging giggly little minis around in dizzying circles. But I couldn't imagine myself mustering the same enthusiasm. I couldn't imagine wanting to.

"It's just not the right time yet," I told Sam over and over again. "Plus, I'm too stressed out with everything that's happening with my parents right now."

"You can't keep putting your life on hold because your parents are going through a rough time," he'd argue. "And honestly, babe, I think you're using your parents' current situation as another excuse to put off having kids."

"No!" I insisted, which was a lie.

The whole first half of 2013 was dominated by this carousel of baby fights and parent worries, anxieties and tempers bobbing like tired, wooden horses. Then Sam and I each started new jobs, and we agreed that, of course, it would be a bad time to try for a baby. Of course. Of *course*. Let's get settled in at work.

Work for me was as a writer at a streaming internet radio company with hella rad coworkers who wore obscure band T-shirts and said things like "hella rad." Sam started as a businessy businessperson at an internet search company that— Fine. Google. Sam got a job at Google. He's going to be mortified by the description "businessy businessperson," but I sincerely did not and still do not understand his job; just that he rode a controversial shuttle bus down to a campus where some of the smartest people in the world played volleyball in between meetings about eyeglasses that can order pizza for you.

My dad was thrilled by these developments, because he thought it meant he had a direct line to his own personal IT helpdesk and music director, that he could call Sam up for computer triage, or call me with music requests, the way you might dial up a radio DJ on a Saturday night and dedicate a song to your best girl.

Only he'd dial me up in the middle of a Tuesday.

"Can you play some Brubeck for me?" he'd ask as soon as I answered.

"*You* can," I'd say in hushed tones, crouched over my cell phone in my cubicle while a Nerf war or freestyle rap session or mindful yoga push-ups session ensued somewhere in the immediate vicinity. "You can type in whatever song or artist you want to hear, and it will play."

"I can?"

"*Yes.* I told you that *yesterday.* Can you please not call during the day unless it's an emergency? That's why I pick up the phone, you know. In case it's an emergency."

"Sure, honey, sorry about that."

But he kept calling. And I kept answering, just in case he had a pressing job search question. I wanted to be available for him, and my coworkers didn't seem to mind. Plus, it was easy to slip into the A-hole.

The company I worked for had a pretty slick setup. Organic snacks everywhere, candy-colored wallpaper, conference rooms designed to look like the bottom of a swimming pool, that kind of thing. One of the kitchens featured the word "radio" cut out in the wall, with a comfy upholstered booth and TV monitor nestled into each letter. We called them the [letter]-holes. The R-hole was the coziest and my favorite, the O-hole was large and airy and good for spreading out with complicated condiments. The A-hole was the butt of many jokes.

One day, I was running hella late for a rad meeting when Dad called again. I declined the call. He called again. And again. Finally, I ducked into a stairwell and answered.

"Dad, I can't talk right now, I—"

"Google is broken!" he screamed at me. "You have to tell Sam."

I laughed, thinking he was kidding. But the laughing only made him madder.

"Sam needs to call someone!" He was yelling now. "I can't get to my fucking email!"

Whoa.

"Dad," I said, taken aback by the f-bomb, "calm down. I promise you that Google is not broken." Oh my god, what was wrong with him? He sounded like his house was on fire. Like he was the one who'd set it.

"Put Sam on the phone!" he snapped. "He needs to tell someone. People rely on Google, even though they're just criminals out to steal your fucking identity."

"Okay, Dad," I said, trying to sound calm for the sake of any eavesdropping coworkers. "Are you looking at your computer right now? Is it on?"

"Yes, I'm looking at my goddamned computer!" he screamed. I hadn't heard him this angry in years. It reminded me of *Chuck Berry's Golden Hits*, and the smack of that lady's face against the brick fireplace. "Nothing's happening."

"Okay. Can you be really specific with me? When you say 'Nothing's happening,' do you mean you're looking at a blank screen? Or have you tried to open your browser and it's not loading? What happens when you try to get online?"

"Nothing fucking happens!" he yelled.

"Dad. I say this *every time*. When you say that *nothing happens*, it doesn't help me understand. I need you to describe to me exactly—"

He hung up.

My phone rang again almost immediately. Mom.

"Sorry about Dad," she said, sounding easy-breezy, like she was trying to smooth things over. "He's just frustrated because Google's broken."

"*Mom*," I said, "what's going *on* with him?

"*Google* is *not broken. And*, I'm at *work*," I continued. "You guys can't just keep calling me all day with whatever the computer problem of the minute is."

Mom got huffy, then *she* hung up on me, and I pulled it together to finally rush off to my meeting about Mumford and Sons.

I had three voicemails by the end of the meeting, from a calmer Dad. He said he was sorry, that he'd been upset because he'd had an idea to write some children's books; collections of the bedtime stories he'd told to me and my brother when we were kids. He'd been inspired by my brother's daughter, LaVera, whom Dad called "La Very Best."

Dad did make up some killer bedtime stories. My favorite was about a milkman who accidentally delivers the wrong flavor to an allergic witch (banana milk instead of chocolate), who retaliates by turning him into a frog. Eventually, the milkman/frog gets ahold of the witch's magic wand, turns her into a fly, and eats her.

Maybe he was abandoning "The Naughty Bride" manuscript, and we'd never talk about it again. What a relief.

"I love this, Dad," I said when I called him back. "What can I do?"

"I'm going to send you the stories that I remember," he said, "plus an idea for a cookbook that I'm going to do with Mom: 'Reindeer Bellybutton Pudding.' It'll be funny recipes for kids."

"Sounds great," I said. "I'll keep an eye out."

Dad did email me the list of bedtime story titles and plot points that he could remember, along with an attached list of other book ideas. I assumed it was other children's books, but:

- Sex After 30
- The Clown Kama Sutra
- My Daily Sex Planner
- Je T'emp: A Lover's Guide to One-Date Romance
  - The awkward first 10 minutes
  - Somebody tell a joke, for godsakes
  - The Road to Hell: When it becomes obvious you're from different planets
  - 10 strategies for making an early exit
  - Weighing the Sex Factor: 3 drinks into it and you're thinking, "It has been a long time..."
  - Your Place, Their Place, or the First Patch of Grass You Encounter?
- Feeling Yourself Up: How to Perform Emotional Plastic Surgery While Your Date Waits in the Car
  - You and your feelings
  - Painting your emotional portrait
  - Interpreting your emotional portrait
  - You and your body
  - Getting your friends to feel you up
- The Sex Diet: Fuck Your Way Thin in 30 Days

There was another attached document called "Condo." Mortgage info? Nope; a full manuscript for a book called "Coming Soon: The Official Condom User's Handbook."

Six Steps to Putting on a Condom

Step 1: Practice, practice, practice

Putting on a condom requires surgical precision. You can't just rip it open with your teeth like a savage animal (it is a turn on, but it tastes like hell) and jam it on Willy nilly. Practice every night at home by rolling condoms onto simple household objects of different shapes and sizes to simulate various states of arousal. When you can bag a popsicle before it melts, a banana, a quart of milk, a lava lamp, a vacuum cleaner hose, a frozen turkey, and a fussy cat, you're ready to move to step 2.

Step 2: Assemble a condom accessory kit...

....that includes small scissors for clipping open the condom foil package, a bandaid for patching up sidewall blowouts, and a shiny trinket to divert your partner's attention from the spurting blood when you forget to drop the scissors before attempting to apply the condom.

Step 3:

Unzip your trousers.

Step 4:

Reach into your trousers and attempt to locate your little soldier.

Step 5:

Look at your partner with soft, pleading eyes and ask, "Would you help me find my little soldier? I think he's asleep at his post."

Step 6:

Lay back while your partner impatiently yanks the condom from your hand, spanks your little soldier, expertly snaps the condom on, and goes to town.

The following week I got a package from my prolific father that contained printouts of his manuscripts for "Reindeer Belly-button Pudding," and another children's story called "The Bully on the Bridge" that was really just the classic story "Three Billy Goats Gruff" with a few details changed. At the bottom of the manuscript pile was something called "Sex After 30," to which he'd paper-clipped a black-and-white cartoon of two people acrobatically entwined in what can best be described as doing the nastiest, most flexible nasty.

I called my mother.

"Okay," I said. "I know we've never really talked about Dad's old books. The, um, sex ones." I had to practically whisper "sex," not only because I was sitting at my desk, surrounded by coworkers who'd gathered to watch a YouTube video of fainting goats, but because I'd never said the word "sex" to my mother before.

But my mom *laughed*. The woman who once gave me a rock-hard NO on the Bon Jovi album *Slippery When Wet* because it included a song called "Social Disease."

"Oh yeah!" she said, like this conversation topic was as worn and comfortable as my father's armchair. "The family business!"

"So, you know that I know about them," I said.

"Sure."

"And you know that he's writing new ones."

"Isn't it great?" she asked.

"I…guess? But you don't think it's weird that his sex books were this big, gross secret my whole life, but then out of nowhere he's just casually throwing out ideas for wedding night fucking—"

"Sara! Don't talk like that."

We argued for a while. I said it was weird that she seemed more upset that I'd said "fucking" than that my father was sending me books about and pictures of fucking. She countered that he was finally just being himself around me, and that maybe it was a compliment, or a sign that he finally saw me as a peer. Or maybe he was just too stressed out and tired to keep up the charade of self-censorship.

"You kids are so hard on me," she said, dropping the act, sounding tired. "We're running out of money; we're doing the best we can. Dad's been trying to get a job; he can't get a job."

"I don't think he's going to get a job," I said, trying not to panic about this new information, that my parents were barreling toward broke.

"I know that," she said. "Do you think he wants to hear it? He's depressed. He doesn't understand the computer. He feels old."

"Something's going on with him," I said. "The computer thing, it's crazy. I can't handle it."

"Try living with it."

"I don't want to."

"Well," my mom said, "*I* don't have a choice."

"What are you going to do?" I asked.

"I'm going to help him start the business," she said. "Books,

T-shirts. Those kid stories he used to tell you. He loved telling those stories; he was so happy that you were going to help him write them down. Are you still going to?"

"Mom."

"It'll be great," she said. "Between the books and T-shirts and his freelance gig, we'll be fine. Oh, here he is, he's dying to talk to you."

"Mom, I can't—"

"I?" she called out. "Sara's on the phone! Hold on, Sar. Here he is. Hold on, he's going to pick up the cordless so we can both talk to you."

"Hi, honey," Dad said. "Did Mom tell you the news? *Games You Can Play with Your Pussy* is number one!"

I took a beat—or maybe seven beats, who can remember how long it takes to reconcile your father's avoidance with his newfound casual breeziness about the word "pussy"?

"What do you mean, Dad?" I finally asked.

He told me that one of his old friends had discovered, and forwarded, an article on the internet, a list of "The 40 Worst Book Titles of All Time." And *Games You Can Play with Your Pussy* was number one.

"It's got over a million views!" he said.

I did a quick search and there it was, on a random viral clickbait website based in Lithuania.

"Um, wow," I said. "Wow. I wonder how they found this?"

"That book is very famous," my mom cut in.

"It paid for college!" Dad said.

"Well," Mom said, "it paid the mortgage on our first house."

"Same thing," Dad said dismissively. "Listen," he continued, "I've been talking to my guy about options for getting it reprinted so we can put it up on Amazon."

" ... Okay."

"And I want to get moving on the other sex books. Are you still okay to help me out with that?"

"*No!*" I blurted loudly, and a few of my coworkers turned away from the goat/Taylor Swift mashup video they'd moved on to, and stared.

Why couldn't my dad understand that talking about sex with him felt so uncomfortable? He was the one who'd set me up to avoid anything sexual at all costs, from the plug-pulling to the uck, feh–ing to that teenage "dreaded ovulation" conversation that had ended with birth control pills and history's most tortured silence. I guess this shouldn't have been such a big deal. I was an adult. Adults talk about sex with other adults, sometimes even comfortably.

But still, it confused me that Dad was suddenly breaking his own conversation rules. Plus, fathers and daughters talking about sex just felt wrong.

I mouthed an apology to my eavesdropping coworkers and lowered my voice. "I've never been okay with, um, *sex* books, Dad," I said. "But I'd love to help you with the kids' books. Is that okay?"

"I understand, honey," Dad said, and promised to send me his latest version of "Reindeer Bellybutton Pudding," plus some other stories he was working on.

He did! It was freaking adorable, and I was so relieved:

Reindeer Bellybutton Pudding

Make your own Xmas Treats for Santa. Pick one from column A , one from Column B and one from column C

A	B	C
Before Dessert		
Barbequed	Monkey	With crackers
Red speckled	Woodpecker	Stew
Un-pumpkin	Meatloaf	With chopsticks
Chocolate	Ants	More than a few
Chicken soup	brimming with knuckles	And noodles
Great mounds	Of potatoes	With cheese
Antelope	antlers	You dip into butter
Red licorice	whips	Thick as trees
The finest American	Root beer	I think you should have one or two
Dessert		
Reindeer	Belly button	Pudding
Three-layer	Elf nose	Pie
Then you could take	A red flannel cake	With blue icing and give it a try
Peppermint	sundaes	with fudge sauce
A wheelbarrow	Full of	Ice cream

Cute, I thought. *I can get behind this, even though "barbecued monkey with crackers" is a little weird and gross.*

But it got weirder. And grosser. Because the other attachment was a new version of "The Naughty Bride," with an illustration of a woman grinding her groom's sausage, reverse-cowgirl-style.

"How is he *sending* these *emails*?!" I moaned to Sam. "He thinks *Google* can *break*, but he figured out how to email me *dick pics*? Not *his* dick," I added quickly.

But the "clueless old man" line felt like tragic pigeon puttering, and it stuck with me. I just kept imagining my father old and sad and aimless in a French apartment, and it sent me over the edge.

As it turns out, Mom felt similarly. Even though she played along with the excitement about *Games You Can Play with Your Pussy* and the "family business" of dog books and sex guides, she called my father's doctor and made an appointment to get his brain checked out. I was so, so glad to be on the same page as her. It made me feel less crazy, less alone in my distress over Dad's about-face, from sexless to shameless.

Fri, April 18, 2014

Dad had his appointment today. It was 2 hours long. They gave him some neurological tests and he said that he didn't do well on some stuff, but did fine on other stuff. I think we will all agree that there is definitely something going on and maybe now we will get some help.

Try not to read between the lines. My feeling is this...yes, there is something going on, but I do not feel that it is anything that can't be helped. I feel that once we get a diagnosis, he will be put on medication. It didn't even occur to me that maybe he might be depressed...that in itself would explain a whole lot. He doesn't do well being alone...sounds funny because he is a man who hates interacting with people, I am NOT scared...concerned, yes, scared, no. I am so positive that help is so close and we will keep pushing until we get answers. I will go to the next appointment and ask a lot of questions. There is no need for you to come home and you and Sam are NOT to interrupt your lives. That is extremely important to us. Things are okay and I expect to be able to handle everything here okay...if I can't or there is any decision to be made, I will consult you.

You are a wonderful daughter and I am the lucky mother to have you. You will make a very wise and wonderful mom someday.

Love, Mom

Mom's line about Sam and I not interrupting our lives—it moved me.

What if I have kids, I thought, *and it's too late? What if by then, Dad's too old to enjoy them, or even meet them?* I made a teary call to my OB/GYN's office and scheduled an appointment to talk about maybe possibly going off birth control, and maybe possibly, but probably not, trying to get pregnant. I wondered if Sam would be disappointed to learn that it was my sad love for my lost father that inspired me to want to try for a kid, and not my happy love for my rock-solid husband. Or if the reason wouldn't matter. Or if I should even tell him. I opted for that last one.

I went off birth control, and a few months later, soaping up in the shower, I looked down and noticed that my left breast was snaked with purple veins. It looked like the throbbing forehead of a sci-fi villain whose world-domination initiative was *not* going according to plan.

And I just *knew*.

It made sense. We'd gone to LA the previous weekend for a friend's fancy beach wedding, and on the way down I'd cried uncontrollably at the in-flight safety video, which featured dozens of beautiful people singing and dancing about emergency floatation devices. They were so good; it was so good. "What an incredible opportunity for artists," I'd sobbed to the stranger in the aisle seat next to me, and felt moved to double-check my seat belt.

Out of the shower, I grabbed one of the pregnancy tests we'd bought in bulk at Costco and peed on it.

Positive.

I peed on another. I peed on three more.

Positive. Positive positive positive.

My doctor's office gave me a same-day urgent care appointment, and I rushed in with all of those traitorous little sticks in a ziplock bag. When I plunked it down in the exam room and asked if I could possibly be pregnant, the nurse practitioner thought I was joking. I insisted on a blood test.

Those results took two weeks, and I mostly spent them hiding out in the office kitchen booths and dreading confirmation of what was already cooking away in my body. I wasn't ready. It happened so fast. How the fuck did it happen so fast? I was years into my thirties—my exponentially shriveling uterus was supposed to be en route to jerky status.

A nurse finally called with the unequivocally positive results and I sat there, completely fucked, in the A-hole.

Sam was over the moon.

When we told my parents, my mom cried and laughed—
Ha! Ha! Ha!—Dad did his singular *ha!* Then he sent me an
email with six outlines for children's stories, plus a blank Word
document called "Cat Picnic."

My mom sent me a separate email.

Chapter 11

THE BEST WE CAN

June 27, 2014

Dear Sara,

Last night I thought about what I would say and decided that it is better to be honest and upfront so that, together we can all make some decisions.

Yesterday we had a meeting with the doctor. Dad has Alzheimer's disease.......MODERATE. He has been put on a medication that will help to stabilize him for about 1 1/2 years. He will not get better, but the point is to keep him stable. The creative part of his brain still functions rather well, so it will be crucial to get him writing. The most important thing is to keep him engaged, so I ask each of you to send him an e-mail once in awhile. He looks for mail everyday. Send slow mail when you can...cards, etc.

We will try to stop the progression for as long as we can. He is depending on all of us to be upbeat and supportive.

We are fine. Had the few tears and now are determined to make life the best that we can.

I love you both. I am so thankful for two wonderful children and I know that you guys are always there for us.

Love, Mom

Part III
After

Chapter 12

THE DREAM GORILLA

Until June 27, 2014, the hardest thing I'd ever read was the darkly funny Russian satire *The Master and Margarita*. I didn't even read it, actually, just tried to. It was one of my dad's favorite books, which seemed so out of character for him, but I guess his character has taken twists and turns for much of my life.

I learned about Dad's passion for *The Master and Margarita* when I was in my early twenties, after I called him to cry about an adult ed writing class I'd started, then immediately dropped out of. To be honest, I'm not a terribly sophisticated reader. I don't get poetry; I need CliffsNotes for Shakespeare. The class was at Harvard, which is a terrible school to spend money on if you're an unsophisticated reader. So, a heads-up on that.

The professor started class by asking each of us to name our favorite book, and when it was my turn I said *Bridget Jones's Diary*. The woman next to me snorted, and said, "Well. *I* prefer works of Russian literature, although *never* in the winter."

Actually, she may have said, "but *only* in the winter." I can't remember exactly, though either answer makes both perfect sense and no sense at all. Maybe if I *were* a terribly sophisticated reader, I'd have gotten the joke or gotten that she was absolutely not joking about this thing, or anything.

I didn't even wait for the class to end, just got right up and walked right out, feeling so ridiculous, and clueless. This was "Johnny B. Goode" all over again, only worse, because little kids make fun of you and then move on. The Russian literature winter woman is probably *still* laughing about me to her friends, nearly two decades later. I bear her no ill will. I hope she's found a Siberian snow cave stocked with Celexa, and someone to share it with.

"*Bridget Jones's Diary*," I muttered to myself as I hoofed it outside into a crisp Cambridge evening, and started to cry. "*Bridget Jones's Diary*. Jesus Christ. You ridiculous asshole."

I crossed Harvard Yard as quickly as I could, eager to put as much space between me and my humiliation as possible. (Before I go any further, if your brain just went to "Pahk ya cah in Hahvahd Yahd!" stop. You can't park there, man. It's grass.) And I called my dad, of course. He'd laughed at me, but not unkindly, then told me about *The Master and Margarita*, and that if I wanted to read some Russian literature, I should start there. I headed straight to one of his favorite bookstores, the Harvard Coop, and very proudly asked a bored-looking student employee to point me toward the classic Russian literature section, please.

"I think you just mean 'classics,'" he yawned, gesturing limply in the general direction of, you know, books.

I wanted to love *The Master and Margarita*, so I could finally have a book that I could openly, unsqueamishly talk about with my father. It's a magical realism celebration of naked flying women and giant cats that can talk. I mean, this is what I've gleaned from internet searches. I couldn't get through the first chapter. Here I'd like to once again apologize to college.

Anyway, *The Master and Margarita* was the hardest thing I'd ever read, until that devastating email from my mom that foreshadowed my dad's cause of death.

At first I was pissed and hurt that she'd revealed such earth-shattering information in an email instead of calling to tell me voice-to-voice, mother-to-daughter. *And* that she sent it in the middle of my workday. I read it right as I was headed into a meeting about a concert my company was sponsoring, and I didn't have time to collect myself before getting into a heated discussion with some audio producers over whether the script for a fifteen-second promo I was writing should end with "Tap the ad to get started," or "Tap the ad to get things started."

"We want people to engage with the ad when they're listening on their phones," argued a man with a cheek piercing and a real attitude, if you ask me. "To tap on the ad so it will click through to our website and they can get things started."

"But what are the *things* we want them to get started on?"

"Buying tickets to the show."

"But 'things' doesn't mean anything."

"It means 'Buy tickets.'"

"But why don't we just *say that*?"

"Because we don't want it to *seem* like we want them to buy tickets."

My coworkers and I argued about things, and "things," for half an hour, and I ultimately emerged victorious but disproportionately crazy mad. Like, foaming at the A-hole. *It's that email's fault I'm this upset*, I reasoned, *and my mother's. Who sends an* email *about something so serious?*

Emboldened by my raw power to overrule a roomful of shaggy men, I marched into an empty Simon and Garfunkel–themed conference room so I could call my mother and bully her into the ultimate Alterman nightmare: difficult conversation. I would demand an explanation as to why she'd communicated the most important information of our lives in a ninety-word email. I would grill her about this diagnosis, and the plan for treatment, and what she was trying to accomplish with an all-caps "MODERATE," and the insanity of a seven-period ellipsis.

But then I thought, *Well shit. I don't want to talk about this either.*

And "moderate," well. Unlike "things," it changed a lot about that horrible sentence: "Dad has Alzheimer's disease." Like, "No big deal! No worries for now!" The all-caps were meant to emphasize the no-big-deal-ness. She didn't want it to seem like she was falling apart.

I did call Mom, but only to tell her that I loved her, and that everything would be fine, and that I'd fly home so we could meet with Dad's doctor together to figure out what to do and expect between now and whenever MODERATE evolved to VERY SERIOUS.

A few weeks later I was back in Massachusetts. I took the same old plane to the trains to the station by the sea, where Dad waited for me on the train platform as usual, shivering in his worn leather jacket, even though it was July. He offered me a small Dunkin' Donuts coffee, so piping hot that the cup scalded my hand.

"Ouch!" I said, nearly dropping it. "Jeez, Dad, it's the middle of summer, you didn't want iced?"

"Iced," he scoffed, grabbing the handle of my suitcase. "Iced is for wussies."

"Well, is it decaf?"

"Decaf? Decaf is for wussies."

"Totally," I said. "But it's also better for the baby."

"Whose baby?" he asked. I held my breath to see if he was kidding, and realized that I had no idea what Alzheimer's really looked like, or how it worked. My knowledge of dementia was secondhand, limited to whatever interpretations I'd seen on TV or in movies, and could generally be boiled down to: batty relative gives up on pants and hairbrushes; rambles about long-lost loves, hateful children, "the war."

But then Dad smiled, and said, to my massive relief, "Your baby's already calling the shots. Now you know the secret to parenting. Just surrender to your children's every whim, and hope they remember your sacrifices when the time comes to choose a nursing home."

I wrapped the hem of my long maternity T-shirt around the scalding cardboard coffee cup, and Dad rolled my suitcase as we walked down to the parking lot, chatting so comfortably about nonsense that I forgot why I was home.

"Why do you think the small cups are cardboard?" I asked him.

"Hmmm?" Dad asked.

"Dunks," I said. "The small cups are cardboard and have flat lids, but all of the other sizes are Styrofoam, with that big domed lid. Why do you think that is?"

"Ha," he said. "You know, I never noticed that before. I bet Mom knows. Ask her, she's right there."

"She's—oh!" I said, as we arrived at the car and I saw that my mom was in the driver's seat. "Mom...drove?"

"Hi, Sary!" my mom said, rolling down her window. Callie the dog immediately scrambled into Mom's lap and from there tried to jump out of the car, desperate to lick and smell the airplane flavors on my face. Mom threw her arms around Callie's wiggling butt just in time. "That's a good girl," she said. "That's Mama's good girl. She's just excited to see you! All

morning long I'd say to her, 'Callie, Sara's coming!' and she'd just
go wild."

"You *drove*, Mom?" I said incredulously, reaching out to pat
Callie's head.

Mom clenched her teeth and shot me a *Cool it!!* kind of look,
and I could tell immediately—though a smidge too late—that I'd
hit a sore subject. My father always drove. Where we were going,
how long it would take us to get there, that was irrelevant. Dad
drove; Mom navigated. When we were kids, Dan and I scooted
as far away from each other in the backseat as humanly possible,
like each of us thought the other smelled like butts, or trouble, or
butt trouble. These days, absent human children, Callie the dog
child stood with her hind legs in the backseat and her front paws
on the console, panting expectantly in between chin scratches
and treats of peanut butter sandwich crackers.

As far as I knew, it had been nearly twenty years since my
father had been a passenger in his own car: 1996. The year I got
my learner's permit, and he taught me how to drive.

I tried to keep my face neutral as I handed Dad my coffee
cup and grabbed my suitcase to put in the trunk, while he
climbed slowly into the passenger seat and fumbled around with
the seat belt.

"There it is, I'm sorry," he said as the buckle finally clicked
into place. "I'm used to coming at it from the other side."

Mom looked at me in the rearview mirror, shooting me that
same silent plea to act like I thought Dad riding shotgun was,
like, totally casual and normal.

So, I did. Beyond the driving, I tried to pretend that *everything* was normal. I said nothing about the little stickers and
Post-its I found all over the house, explaining how to use the
remote control, or which light switches controlled which lights.

I ignored the red and green dots that color-coded the on/off buttons on the coffeemaker and the thermostat.

After dinner that night, my father disappeared into the basement to play solitaire on his computer. It was my first moment alone with my mother since the diagnosis—or The Diagnosis, I guess—and it felt rushed and hushed, like I needed to get all of my questions answered before Dad came upstairs to discover what I was sneakily up to, like the way it always felt when I was a kid, stealing secret moments with his books.

"What's the deal?" I whispered to Mom as I helped her clear the table, which I most certainly did, and am definitely not just painting myself as a dutiful table-clearing daughter. "He's not driving now?"

"Doctor's orders," Mom said. "And not a moment too soon. He's been driving into the oncoming lanes of traffic, and thank God the doctor said something."

"Didn't *you* say something?!"

"Well, I tried, Sar, but he wouldn't listen to me."

"*Mom.* You could just refuse to get in the car."

She ignored me and plugged in an electric teakettle, which was weird. For as long as I could remember, my parents made their after-dinner tea with amaretto using a sturdy metal kettle that whistled louder than a steam train.

"You've gone electric?" I asked.

"I had to," she said. "Whenever Dad tries to use the stove he cranks the burner up full blast without igniting the pilot. He keeps filling the house with gas. I had to hide all of the matches, just in case."

This was all so hard to hear, to swallow, to accept, to handle. Hard to . . . everything. I felt like a garbage person, for being outrageously annoyed by Dad's computer problems, his endless job search, for the behavior I'd written off as bumbling old-man-itis. This whole time his brain had been fighting itself, and I hadn't noticed. What kind of daughter doesn't notice that?

A few days later, I asked Dad's doctor, Dr. G., a version of that same question.

Dr. G. was a perfectly nice and competent man who specialized in elder care and weight loss, which seemed strangely disconnected and also a strange match for my father's neurological needs. But Mom and Dad felt comfortable with him, so I was willing to keep an open mind. He was happy to have me at the appointment and said that he always welcomed adult children into the conversation.

"Who are you calling an adult child?" Dad joked. He was sitting on an exam table, startling himself every time he shifted positions and the table paper crumpled. Mom stood next to him, holding his hand, while I sat on a tiny stool in the corner and tried to make myself as small as possible, even though I wanted to rise up and roar at this random doctor for daring to diagnose my dad with dementia.

Doctor dared diagnose Dad's dementia.

It was the kind of clever alliteration my father ate with a spoon. I started to say it out loud, but Dr. G. cut me off, unaware.

"How are you feeling today, Ira?" he asked, clicking a pen open, which startled my father again.

"Good," Dad said, "I feel good. Hungry."

Dr. G. made a note on a thick yellow legal pad. "That's good," he said.

He and my parents talked for a while about medication and routine and diet and Dad's general day-to-day mood and habits. Dr. G. took copious notes. Dad wouldn't look at me. He wouldn't even say "Alzheimer's," he just kept referring to "my condition."

Can I have a job with my condition? What else can we do about my condition? Why can't I drive, is it because of my condition?

The doctor assured my father that the medication he'd prescribed, Namenda, was the best option available to dementia patients.

"Just let me know if you get too constipated," he said, closing his pen with another click. All of us Altermans looked at the floor. We are not bathroom-talk people. Which, at this point, should not come as a surprise.

My mom recovered from her embarrassment first, and thanked Dr. G. for his time. She took Dad gently by the arm to lead him out to the waiting room. I stayed behind.

"Can I talk to you for a minute?" I asked Dr. G.

"Of course," he said, and clicked his pen back open.

"I'll be right out," I said to Mom, and then I closed the door.

"What's really going on?" I asked.

Dr. G. raised an eyebrow. "What do you mean?"

"I mean, I think my parents are trying to hide stuff from me."

"How so? They seem like they're being pretty transparent."

"I don't know." I felt so exasperated and tired. "My mom told me the diagnosis in an email. She said it's just moderate Alzheimer's and he's going to be stable for at least a year and a half."

"That's right," Dr. G. said.

"And he keeps talking about getting a job. And starting a 'family business' doing, um, some writing. But it's just bullshit, you know? I'm sorry to swear. I'm just—"

"Frustrated," Dr. G. said. "And scared for your dad. I understand. Part of my method is to work with adult children in managing their parents' treatment plan and care."

"Who are you calling an adult child?" I said weakly, trying to echo my father's joke but getting the tone all wrong.

Dr. G. ignored it. "Sometimes it's hard for parents to fold their children into a treatment plan," he continued, "especially if they have a tendency to protect you from difficult or painful information."

I nodded.

"Your father needs to stay optimistic," Dr. G. continued. "It's true that he won't get a job. Even if he does, it's not appropriate or, probably, even possible for him to work anymore. But as long as *looking* for a job isn't causing him too much stress, it's a good activity."

"It's causing everyone stress," I said. "He's been looking for a job for years; it's brutal. It's like we're all screaming into empty closets, you know? Just, like, throwing résumés into a black hole."

Dr. G. nodded. "Then let's discourage him from doing that anymore," he said.

"Do you think I should move home?" I asked. "To take care of him?"

"Where do you live?"

"San Francisco."

"And you have a husband there? A job? And your mom told me you're expecting a baby, congratulations."

Oh, right. Shit, I'd completely forgotten about my own pregnancy. Great. A terrible daughter and, already, a terrible mother.

"Thanks," I said. "But, you know, none of that means that I can't come back here to help them. My husband's from Massachusetts too; I'm sure we could figure it out."

"I don't think that's necessary right now," Dr. G. said. "Your dad is stable."

"But when would it be necessary? How long do I have before he needs me to be here?"

Dr. G. sighed. He must have had this conversation dozens of times, with dozens of helpless adult children. "Look," he said gently, "I'm going to be frank with you. There's no predicting what can happen. We've got your dad on one of the more effective medications that are available, but it's not a cure. Just a treatment. It can help slow the disease's progression, but I want to be clear that he is not going to get better. He'll have good days and bad days, and eventually, just bad days."

I took a second, or maybe it was an hour, to absorb all of that. "Right," I said, swallowing. "Yeah. Okay. It's just…this is all happening really fast."

"I know it seems that way," he said, "but based on everything your mother's told me about Ira's ongoing symptoms, I think the disease began to emerge a few years ago, but nobody caught it. It's not uncommon for early symptoms of dementia to go unnoticed."

"Like what?" I asked. "What symptoms? That's what's so weird, he seemed totally normal."

"Dementia symptoms can present in very subtle ways," Dr. G. said. "A lot of times, people chalk them up to old age. It's not like what you see in the movies or on television. Usually the first thing people notice is poor driving, which happens because of vision changes, or feelings of disorientation, or difficulties with spatial awareness. Your dad might make impulsive financial decisions, or seem confused about things that he used to understand clearly. He might seem confused in general. He might behave inappropriately, or say inappropriate things, without even realizing that he's making people uncomfortable."

I thought of the computer woes and the Google fury, the curb-jumping and the condo-buying. The sex talks, and books, and pictures. I thought of my wedding dress. I thought of "The

Naughty Bride." I thought of the *Amour* pigeon, that sad little French rat with wings.

"Your dad is scared," Dr. G. said. "Alzheimer's is a scary thing. He knows the road he's headed down, and there's nothing anybody can do to change course. The medications can only stabilize him. There's no cure. Yet."

The doctor kept throwing information at me. It was just as well. I couldn't speak. "If you want to help him," he said, "have a long talk with your parents about their long-term plans. What kind of care would they like to procure for your dad? What can they afford? What does he want to do in an emergency? Who does he want to make decisions for him, once he can't make them for himself?"

"I have no idea," I said.

"Start there. And in the meantime, he needs to have immediate goals to focus on, a sense of purpose. You mentioned a family business. Does he have any passions?"

I thought of "Sex After 40," and *Games You Can Play with Your Pussy*, and all of those unfinished books that Dad wanted me to help him finish.

"He has passions," I said.

———

When I was born, on an unseasonably warm evening in early November, my father was a well-meaning disaster; a sheepish bull in a hospital gift shop. He called my mom's obstetrician at the first signs of her labor, but furiously cut the call off after less than a minute, bellowing about what an incoherent moron their obstetrician was, and how such a dimwit couldn't be trusted to deliver a pizza, much less my parents' child. Mom calmly took the receiver from his hand, turned it around, and placed it back in its cradle. He'd been speaking into the end for listening and listening to the end for speaking. I'm sure those are not technical terms.

En route to the hospital, my parents came to a railroad crossing just as the warning lights started to flash. Powerless to stop the descending gate, my desperate dad jumped out of the car and started pleading with the train to stop, or to hurry up, either one, just pick one, quickly, so he could pass through. *My wife's having a baby, goddamnit!* he screamed.

"It was so funny," Mom said. "Nobody could hear him. And even if they could, what, was the train just going to stop, and back up? Dad was out of his mind, so worried that something would go wrong. Then, seventeen hours later, at 5:55 in the evening, you were born, all pink and white."

I'd heard that story, and other stories from the night I was born, dozens of times. But this time I, an adult child, lay with my head in my mama's lap, listening to the story of my birth just a few hours after a doctor told me to start preparing for my daddy's death.

We were on the couch in the honky-tonk condo's living room, talking barely above a whisper. Not that it mattered. Dad was in the basement sipping tea and amaretto by the blue glow of his laptop, lost in another round of solitaire.

"Seventeen hours," I said, shuddering, and reached down to touch my stomach. Three months pregnant. I didn't look very pregnant, but I felt it. Or, at least I felt heavy with extra fluid and goo. And guilt.

"Did it hurt?" I asked, and Mom laughed.

"It was brutal," she said. "I was begging the doctor to knock me out with a baseball bat."

"What about painkillers?"

"I didn't take any."

"Damn," I said, and *Damn*, I thought. *I want any drug anyone will give me. I want two of each of all of the drugs. I want someone to invent new drugs just for me.*

Mom laughed again and said, "And then, after I'd been pushing for hours, with nothing to show for it, your father decided to go out for a hamburger. And Sara"—she snorted—"that man brought it back to my hospital room and started to eat it in front of me. And the smell of it, I'll never forget it: It smelled. So. Good. And I was. So. Hungry. I started crying, and pleading with him for one bite, just please one bite. But they don't let you eat when you're in labor. So Dad just turned around and ate with his back to me."

"That's messed up," I said, like I say every time she tells me this story. This time, though, I could understand her desperation. Lately I'd been having midmeal cravings for the same meal; as in, I'd be eating a breakfast burrito and be struck by an urgent need to eat a breakfast burrito, then have to tell myself—actually speak to myself out loud—*It's okay. Sara. You're already eating a breakfast burrito. Take a deep breath and take another bite. You're doing great.*

"Well, he didn't want to miss anything!" Mom said. "He didn't want to miss you."

"I still think that's crazy."

"Well," she said, stroking my hair, "having a baby makes you crazy. But then, you were here! You came out and they put you right on my chest; you never cried. I was screaming, 'What's wrong with her? Why isn't she crying?' And the doctor said, 'Nothing. She's just happy to be here.' And it's true. You just stuck your hand in your mouth and looked around with these big, curious eyes. And then they gave you to me and you looked at me like, 'Oh! There you are, you found me!'

"Dad took so many pictures. He was getting up on chairs to get different angles. People kept asking me if he was a photographer. He was so in love with you. And then, of course, Dad forgot to put film in the camera." Mom chuckled. "Big surprise."

"What do you mean?" I asked. "Why 'of course'?"

"Oh, you know," Mom said, "Dad's always been kind of forgetful."

My mother has told the story of my birth so often that I know it by heart, even though I always act like and ask questions as though I'm hearing it for the first time. By now I've even memorized her cadence, her one-liners. She's terrific at making jokes sound fresh and spontaneous, even when they're a precisely timed part of the same old script.

But this was the first time she'd ever said that my dad forgot film for his camera because "he's always been kind of forgetful."

"Wait," I said. "Really? He has?"

"Mmm-hmm!" Mom said, and then we were quiet together for a long time. She fell into a rhythm with the hair-petting, and it made me sleepy. While I struggled to stay awake I wondered if maybe, like me, my mother was trying to explain away some of Dad's early Alzheimer's symptoms, so that she could forgive herself for missing them.

I should have said something to her, like that there was nothing to forgive because she'd done nothing wrong, that she's an amazing partner to my dad and that we're all lucky to have her.

But I didn't. I rolled off the couch, kissed my mom's soft cheek, grabbed a spoonful of peanut butter from the kitchen, and went upstairs to bed. I guess it just felt easier to end the night on a known, safe story than to talk about anything new and raw with an unknown ending.

———

Something Dr. G. said really unsettled me, which was that Alz-heimer's doesn't play out like you see in movies or on TV. After Mom sent the diagnosis email, I'd clung to the thinnest shred of comfort; that at least I knew what to expect, because of Ronald Reagan, and Gena Rowlands's character in *The Notebook*, and the hysterically senile Abe Simpson. Dad would be okay for a while, but as his body picked off its own brain cells, he'd spend a decade or two transforming into a baby with gray hair, gray skin, and gray moods, blissfully unaware of his own demise. He'd forget names, forget faces, start wearing flowerpots on his head and living in an attic. He'd start to think that I was my mother, and that my mother was a stranger. He'd talk about nonsense. We'd have to push him around in a wheelchair and spoon-feed rice pudding to him. My father already liked rice pudding, so that part didn't seem like a big deal.

But none of this was going to happen, or maybe some of it would, or maybe different things. There was no knowing. My father *was* scared. He would talk about his "condition" with the same stilted, fakey-funny voice he'd used a billion car rides ago, when he'd had to bring up the "dreaded ovulation," the voice where you can practically hear the finger quotes hanging in the air. *Air quotes, Sara.*

———

When I was five or six, there were a few weeks where I was plagued by terrible nightmares. I can't remember what triggered them, if anything at all. Night after night I'd wake up sweating and have to thunder into my parents' room and vault myself in between them in their bed. I was afraid to close my eyes at night, because I didn't know what was going to happen.

The very scariest dream I had was about a murderer who was terrorizing my town. In the dream, we lived in an old-timey seaside village, with a boardwalk and fried-clam stands, and sandy paths that were lined with low, scratchy bushes.

The murderer disguised himself or herself with a cartoonish cow costume that reminded me of a football team mascot, with an overexaggerated head and dopey arms. There had been dozens of victims, and I decided I'd had it. I staked out the boardwalk until I saw the silly cow lumbering along on two legs. Before I could stop it, NO! The cow slaughtered an innocent girl in front of a saltwater taffy store. Other people looked on, horrified, but I followed him away from the crime scene, down to the beach.

There, I crouched behind a sand dune, waiting for the cow to remove his costume and reveal his human identity. And when he did, the person beneath the cartoonish cow head was...another cow. A cow masquerading as another cow, to do murders.

When I tell the story of that dream now I can hear how ridiculous it is, but at the time there was nothing more terrifying to me than this bizarre reveal, that you can have a completely unpredictable secret beneath the face you show to the world.

Anyway, Dad either had great sympathy for me or was greatly fed up with having his sleep interrupted. The next night, when he came in to tell me a bedtime story, he gave me a small stuffed gorilla with white Albert Einstein fur.

"This isn't a toy," he said as he tucked the white gorilla into bed with me. "This is a very special thing called a dream gorilla."

Dad told me that the special thing about a dream gorilla is that it protects you as you sleep. If you start to have a nightmare, he said, the dream gorilla will show up and grow really big, and scare away the monsters and bad guys, and cows.

It worked. Not forever. I still had, and have, bad dreams from time to time (although nowadays they're mostly related to high school, like it's the end of the year and I realize that there's one math class that I haven't been to all year, and if I fail it, I won't graduate). But the run of nightmares stopped, and when I clutched my dream gorilla and closed my eyes at night, I felt secure, and at peace. Although I still didn't know what was going to happen, I knew I was safe.

What kind of stuffed dream animal can you give to a terrified Alzheimer's patient, so that he can feel secure and at peace? Maybe an elephant? They never forget.

Chapter 13

UPS AND DOWNS

We quickly fell into a routine, to try to keep Dad feeling oriented. My parents took Callie for daily walks that they measured in numbers of "ups" and "downs." They liked taking a trail they'd discovered at the end of a cul-de-sac. It wound through a meadow and down a wooded hill to a conservation area, ultimately spilling into a wide-open field that people used as an off-leash dog park. Beyond the dogs were soccer fields, and beyond those, across a street that may have technically been in New Hampshire, was another hilly meadow with paths mowed through a blanket of tall, swishy grasses and goldenrods. Along the way they'd keep track of the hills they climbed. A good day was four ups and four downs. A bad one was no walk at all.

Dad looked forward to checking the mailbox every day, so I sent him cards, trying to find quirky ones that would make him laugh. The first one featured a hand-drawn orange mustache with "hello." written underneath; then I sent a blue one that read "I am your biggest," followed by a picture of an oscillating fan. There was one with colorful silhouettes of beets and eggplants that read "eat your vegetables," and another with a drawing of two foxes holding hands.

In return he'd send me grateful emails and include lists of new books he wanted us to write together. Some were the same sex books he'd been mentioning for a while, "Sex After 30," and "The Clown Kama Sutra." But he also wanted help with a silly holiday parody called "The Rabbi's Night Before Christmas" and a series of children's books to be called Tell Me a Story, Daddy, which was a collection of the bedtime stories he'd made up for me and Daniel when we were little. He had a million ideas; they were all over the place; *he* sounded all over the place. He wanted to do everything, quickly. I think he was desperate to make progress on his publishing goals while he still had the energy.

Mom begged me to help him. "It would be such a good project for the two of you to bond over," she said. "All he wants to do is write books with you."

"*Why?*" I asked. "He's never even wanted to talk about his old books before, and now he wants to write them?"

"I don't *know*, Sara," Mom said, and she sounded so exasperated with me, and tired of everything. "But could you just go with it? Please?"

I was torn. "I don't know, Mom," I said. "Those books are … a lot for me."

My mother sighed. "I understand," she said, and I could tell she was holding something back.

Finally, she said: "He just sits there in front of the computer all day. Sometimes I think he's just waiting to die."

Those words were a hovering hummingbird, plotting its next move.

"The books and the baby," Mom said. "Those are the things he's looking forward to."

Oh, right, I thought, for the second time. *The baby*.

———

After my mom said that Dad was just waiting to die, I felt responsible for saving him. I decided to help him with whatever books he wanted.

When I told him, he was so excited. Not just that we would be working together, but that we would build my inheritance together, a legacy that I could carry on after he was gone.

"Sure, Dad," I said.

"Do you remember the stories I used to tell you kids?"

"Yeah."

"Could you write out what you remember? Maybe you can start with those, and then I can mail you some stuff."

"Okay, Dad," I said, fully relieved. Maybe my mom talked to him. Maybe he wasn't so far gone that he was immune to reason, to reminders that asking your daughter to cowrite a sex book crossed a boundary that couldn't be uncrossed.

Nope.

A few days later I got a package containing a manila folder, with "Sex After 40" written on the tab. Inside was a printout of a manuscript; the same book he'd asked me to help him blog about a few years earlier. There was also a four-panel illustration from "The Clown Kama Sutra." In each panel, a tiny clown is doing his best to pleasure a fellow merry carny. One panel, captioned "Too much of a good thing," shows the clown's face peering up through the crossed legs of a beach ball–breasted "fat lady." In another, captioned "Excuse me, is this seat taken?" he tries his best to mount her from behind.

Then there was "My Daily Sex Planner" again, the manuscript for a book he'd been mentioning for a few years. This one had several pages of charts where you could record your sexual escapades.

> Who:_____
> When:_____
> What: O/A/V/Ran the table
> Wierd stuff?_____
> Rate your date 1-10

I don't know what "ran the table" means, but it was pretty clear that O was "oral," A was "anal," and V was "vaginal."

Another page, "Weights & Measures," was a place to keep track of your lovers' breasts, listing their name, size, and "distinguishing characteristics." It read "Women's breasts can be big, small, or asymmetrical (different sizes), vary in volume, density, size of nipples, and areolas and where they are placed on the chest—high and round, or sagging."

The last few pages were the "Sex Position Reference Library," and, for lack of a delicate way to say this, it was just pictures of people fucking.

So, not children's books then.

I decided my best approach here was to just screen for and correct typos. Maybe if I took a copyediting approach, and complimented his work, that would be good enough.

With one eye closed—not metaphorically, truly—I took a red pen to the manuscript, starting with the table of contents. I changed "Stud or Dudl?" to "Stud or Dud," removed the 'i' from "My Sex Gioals." I corrected "Wierd" to "Weird," added a legend to the charts, explaining what O, A, and V meant. I'd have to ask my dad about "ran the table." Ugh.

This approach worked pretty well, for a while. I'd shoot Dad a quick *Great job! No notes!* email, or let him know that I'd found some typos, never commenting on the actual material. But then Dad called and said he wanted to know what I knew about sexting, and cybersex, so that he could be up-to-date on all of the sex trends.

"I don't know anything about those things," I said, and he sounded disappointed.

"Oh," he said. "Well, that's okay, honey. Maybe you could ask around to some of your friends?"

"Sure, Dad," I lied. This was so hard. I was trying to be open, and to be less uptight, but Dad's the one who closed me off from all of this sex stuff in the first place.

"Thanks, sweetie," he said happily. "Now, how's that baby?"

By then "that baby" was eighteen weeks along and, according to some pregnancy book that appeared on my desk, it was the size of a sweet potato. There was a whole size/food chart.

Once word got out at work that I was pregnant, a rash of well-meaning friends and coworkers began to leave books on my desk: pregnancy books, parenting books, science-based books, blog-based books, hippie crunchy books based on whispers from the moon. One morning I arrived, wantonly clutching a breakfast burrito, to discover a thick paperback waiting for me on my keyboard: *Ina May's Guide to Child-birth*, by Ina May Gaskin, who, I learned on her website, self-identifies as the nation's leading midwife. I didn't know anything about midwives, so I had no reason not to believe her.

I feel guilty admitting this, but I wasn't very happy to be pregnant. And not just because I was nauseous in new ways, and hairy in new places, but because I still didn't think I wanted to be a mother. My feelings about the whole thing had been overshadowed by my feelings about Dad's diagnosis, and we were all so caught up in trying to keep him feeling safe and secure that I hadn't fully processed that *shit, we're having a baby.* And, shit, I didn't really want to have a baby.

Everyone else in my life was thrilled. My parents wanted every detail of every OB/GYN visit. I told them how we'd heard the baby's heartbeat, a *womp womp womp* that could easily be sampled and used on a German house music track. I told them about the fruit chart, that soon the baby would be as big as a mango, and then a banana, and then a carrot.

"It's a produce section in there!" Dad laughed.

And, of course, I told them we were having a boy.

I'd found out while I was at work, of course, sitting at my desk and writing a :30 ad for yogurt cups. A nurse called to tell me, and I burst into tears. My boss asked why I was crying, and I told her.

"Holy shit!" she said, then, hesitantly, "Is…that…good? You're crying, so I don't know."

"It's good," I said, and it was. Not because I cared which gender the baby was, but because now it felt like I had a real person in there, and not just a blob of indifference.

I slipped out into a stairwell to call Sam, and I could tell that his heart just burst wide open. "I can't wait to meet that guy!" he said, in a way that made "that guy" sound like "That Guy™" so from then on, that's what we called the baby.

Dad started sending me emails with random advice, namely, "Never wake a sleeping baby!" He'd also insert it into nearly every phone conversation we had, and I thought maybe he was making an inside joke, like, pretending we had a catch-phrase. But when I teased him about it, he had no idea what I was talking about. Every time Dad advised me to never wake a sleeping baby, he thought he was telling me for the first time.

Were we starting to really lose him? Dr. G. had said he'd be stable for at least a year and a half, but it had been only a few months since his diagnosis. I thought we had more time. I thought *he* did.

Chapter 14

THE HOMETOWN NOSTALGIA
SEND-OFF TOUR

"I have this amazing idea for you," Mom's latest email began. "You and Dad should take a trip to Perkasie."

Perkasie, Pennsylvania; Dad's hometown.

Mom wrote that Dad had been yearning to go there; he had been talking a lot about his childhood and reminiscing about his family. She thought that maybe he was mentally preparing to start forgetting everyone.

It made sense to me. If I knew for sure that I was going to start losing my memories, I'd want to say good-bye to them too.

I agreed to take Dad and asked if Mom wanted to come too. "No" was her response. "I think you and Dad should go alone. He really would enjoy the company of his daughter. It would be wonderful for the two of you. Callie and I will hang out at home and eat lobster!!"

Translation: Please take him for me. I'm so tired.

A few days before, she'd admitted that Dad was waking up in the middle of the night and starting his daytime routine. He'd shower, eat breakfast, clip Callie's leash on, all around two or three in the morning. Mom had begun setting an alarm for the middle of the night so she could catch him in the act and keep him from leaving the house. She couldn't really sleep and was always on edge, afraid that he would hurt himself or someone else. He was still accidentally filling the house with gas from the stove burners, on a semiregular basis. Mom said she'd stopped wearing slippers and fleece socks around the house, just in case she scuffed them and accidentally made a spark.

My mom badly needed a break, and I was the only person who could give her one. I haven't mentioned Daniel in a while. By this point he was in the Army and deployed on a yearlong tour of duty. I emailed him updates every once in a while, but I didn't want to pile too much onto the stress of being in a literal war zone.

We decided that I'd fly to Boston, rent a car, and drive Dad the five-ish hours out to Perkasie. Dad's brother, Jay, was going to meet us there.

Back on a plane to Boston I went, back on the subway to the train up to the sea. You know the drill by now. My parents picked me up at the train station, as usual; Dad waiting for me on the platform when I disembarked, as usual. He was wearing a windbreaker and clutching two cups of coffee.

"Decaf!" he said, handing me one of the cups and grabbing the handle of my roller bag. "Mom said you have to have decaf. You look great."

"You don't need to take that, Dad," I said, trying to grab the suitcase handle back.

"You're pregnant!" he said. "I can't roll a suitcase for my pregnant daughter?"

"You can," I said. "I'm sorry."

"Mom and Callie are in the car," he said. "How's the baby?"

"I brought new pictures!" I said, and pulled my latest ultrasound photos out of my pocket. They were grainy and kind of spooky;

a footprint of bones and a skeletal hand flung dramatically across a grim-looking skull.

"Pictures?" he asked, looking concerned. "Is the baby born? I thought he wasn't born yet. Did you have the baby?"

"No, Dad," I said. "They're printouts from my last ultrasound."

"Oh. Okay, good. I thought I'd missed the baby."

"I won't let you miss the baby," I said.

When we got home I showed the ultrasound printouts to my parents. "They're kind of grainy," I said, "but you can see the baby's hands and feet."

"He has Sam's big feet!" Mom said, but I don't know why. Sam's feet are pretty average.

"Bigfoot!" Dad said. "Wow. You've got a bigfoot in there. Is he kicking?"

"Definitely."

"Moving around okay?"

"Yup."

"Speaking of moving around," Mom said, "you two should get on the road." Ha. She clearly couldn't wait to have the house to herself. If I were her, I'd probably scuff all over the place in my slippers, sparks be damned.

"Oh yeah, Perkasie!" Dad said. "What's the plan? Are we taking the Pennsylvania Turnpike?"

"Don't know," I said. "I'll just start my GPS once we get in the car."

"Let me print out directions," he said.

"You don't need to— Okay." He was already thundering down the basement stairs to his computer.

Mom and I packed up their car with my father's provisions: two suitcases, two extra jackets, a cooler full of milk, juice, and eggs, three cloth grocery bags stuffed with cinnamon raisin bagels and packets of Sweet'N Low and three full boxes of Trader Joe's O's. The crunchy cardboard cereal he claimed to hate.

"We're only going for four days, Mom," I said. "Does he really need all of this?"

"Just take it," she said. "He needs his routine."

"Three boxes of cereal?"

"Sometimes it's all he'll eat."

"I thought he hated it?"

"He needs the routine."

The car rental center was only a mile away, so just a few minutes later we unloaded and reloaded all of the groceries and suitcases into the tiny trunk of an economy sedan, and Dad and I were on our merry way, to see Perkasie for the last time. I'd been calling this trip the Hometown Nostalgia Send-Off Tour, which captures it, I think. Dad wanted to go and relive warm, happy memories from his childhood before he lost them.

"I brought music!" he said as we pulled out of the parking lot, producing a thick black book of CDs. He flipped through the plastic pages and carefully slipped one out; an experimental jazz mix he'd made and burned to disc, back when he knew how to do that.

"This is one of my favorites," he said, popping it into the CD player.

Silence. I jabbed at the buttons, I turned the stereo on and off. Nothing. I hit eject. It wouldn't come out. The CD had disappeared into the stereo's guts forever. I mean, an experimental jazz mix. Maybe the car was just doing me a favor.

"It's okay, Dad," I said. "We can use my phone to listen."

I plugged it into the car's auxiliary input, but no sound came out. I tried the radio, nothing. Shit.

Dad was distraught. He kept trying to stick his fingers into the CD slot, then he tried his house keys. There was no way I could handle a music-free road trip that was five hours long, so I turned around and went back to the rental office. They gave me a new car, and promised to try to get the CD out. Dad was super upset.

"It's okay, Dad," I said. "If you still have the music files on your computer, I can just burn you another CD."

"Tell them that's my CD," he said. "Make sure they get it out."

"I will."

"It's my CD."

"I know. I promise."

The drive was challenging in ways I hadn't anticipated. Dad asked me again and again and again if we were going to take the Pennsylvania Turnpike, if our driving route would take us anywhere near the Pennsylvania Turnpike, when we were going to get to the Pennsylvania Turnpike. My mother had warned me that some symptoms of Alzheimer's were repetition and fixation, but it was truly a subtle form of torture. What could I say? Dad needed to know about the turnpike, and he'd forgotten that he'd already asked. I tried to be patient, but, to be honest, I wanted to pull the car over and leave him by the side of the road. Just for a few minutes! I'd go back for him. I'm not a monster.

Every ten minutes or so, Dad would pull out a pack of gum, meticulously unwrap a piece, and pop it into his mouth. Then he'd remember, *Oh yeah!* He already had another piece of gum in his mouth. So he'd spit them both back into the wrapper, smush it into a little ball, toss the ball in the cupholder, and start the whole cycle again.

And then there was Dunkin' Donuts. Every time we drove past a Food/Gas/Lodging sign with the holy pink-and-orange

Dunkin' Donuts logo, Dad would cry out like a scurvy-riddled pirate spotting land.

Dunkin' Donuts!

Dunkin' Donuts! Pit stop!

Dunkin' Donuts! Pit stop before we hit the Pennsylvania Turnpike?

We stopped five times so Dad could have French crullers and medium coffees with cream and three Sweet'N Lows. All in all, our five-ish-hour drive took closer to nine.

We finally arrived, way after dark, and only a few minutes before Jay did. Jay is Dad's younger brother, and Dad talked about him with a lot of love. They kept in close touch but rarely saw each other, hadn't lived anywhere near each other since they were children. I hadn't seen Jay since *I* was a child, and I think the last time was at his wedding, in the late '80s. Somewhere there's a photo of me from the reception, standing at the bar, sipping a Coke from a highball glass. Even though my uncle was mostly a stranger to me, I was glad to have him along.

Our Airbnb, a 2,000-square-foot house with three stories and not enough showers, was in a tiny town near Perkasie called Riegelsville. Population: 868. I shuffled Dad inside and got him settled on a couch so I could unload the car. My father was agitated because my GPS route hadn't put us on the Pennsylvania Turnpike.

"We can't be in Pennsylvania!" he protested as I draped a blanket over his skinny legs. "Should you check the route? We didn't take the turnpike."

"We're here, Dad."

I let Jay and Dad have the second-floor bedrooms and claimed the private third floor for myself. There was a living room with a pull-out couch, and a literal water closet at the top of the stairs; just a front-facing toilet and tiny sink shoehorned into what had clearly once been a linen closet. There was no door, just a sheer curtain to shield my dirty business from anyone who poked their head up and around the corner from below. Of course, Dad did just that around five o'clock the next morning, while I was hovering in between asleep and awake while also hovering over the john. "She's pissing!" he called out to nobody. Then he said he was heading out for a walk to look for coffee and antiques.

The baby had dicked around in my guts all night and I'd barely slept. It may have been a dream, but I faintly remembered that Dad had tapped on my door in the middle of the night to ask if I wanted a donut. Where did he think he was going to get donuts before dawn in pastoral Pennsylvania? Same place he thought he was getting coffee and antiques, probably a place that he'd invented, a place that didn't exist.

After I watered the water closet I tried to go back to sleep but remembered that I should probably stop my dad from walking out the door to wander around a strange rural place where there are plenty of trees to hang "Missing: 69-year-old Alzheimer's Patient" posters but not enough people to hang them.

Downstairs, I was relieved to see my dad and my uncle sitting at the dining room table. Jay had made coffee. Dad was eating one of his cinnamon raisin bagels with a knife and fork. "There she is!" He smiled, then stood up from the table and plopped a floppy brown fedora on his head. "Let's roll."

Perkasie is a small and bucolic town in Bucks County, close to other small towns and unincorporated communities with names like Lumberville, Mechanicsville, and Fountainville. There's also Eureka, which I like to imagine as a place where people get their big ideas.

There are nationally registered historic covered bridges in

Perkasie, and honor system roadside farm stands, and a midcentury carousel that, according to their historical society's website, is "a rare example of original Allan Herschell Art Deco style rounding boards and scenery." It was not the original carousel, which was built in 1891 and featured hand-carved horses, but it was the one that my dad and his brothers and friends would ride on before, or maybe after, grabbing sweet treats at the nearby Dairy Queen.

"Well, gentlemen," I began as we loaded ourselves into the car. Somewhere out in the fog, a rooster crowed. "Where should we start our hometown tour?"

Dad said, "Home."

The old Alterman homestead is in South Perkasie, on the corner of Virginia Avenue and East Market Street. It's a squat brick house, with a white storm door that's crowned by a small portico and flanked by two large, stern windows. It reminded me of a disapproving owl, staring down the bridge of its weather-resistant beak.

We parked across the street and got out to creep around.

"Look, I," Jay said, pointing to the side of the house. "Dad's wall is still there."

"My father built that retaining wall by the driveway," Dad explained to me. "God, that thing's still standing. When was that, Jay? What year?"

Jay shrugged. "Nineteen something?" he said.

"Nineteen something," Dad said, and Jay reached out to straighten his brother's hat.

Dad wanted me to take their picture in front of the house, and they shuffled over to stand shoulder to shoulder. "Make sure to get my good side," he said, his face all floppy hat and aging beard.

"Which one is that?" I teased.

"Ha! Neither one of them," he said. "Both of them. I don't know. I'm an old man."

"Say cheese, Dad."

He didn't. But I took the picture, and then he and Jay looked at each other with big, happy grins, like they were sharing a private joke.

"Can we go see the curtains now?" Dad asked.

"Susie!" Jay smiles. "I think she's still there."

"There are curtains named Susie?" I asked.

"Our neighbors," Dad said to me, and pointed down Market Street. "Down there. Three kids. Two boys and a girl." He started walking down the street.

Jay and I followed.

"Three boys and a girl," Jay said, "or maybe one boy? You know, Ira, I can't remember."

"Your grandmother asked your grandfather to have some curtains made," Dad called back to me. "He was a manager at a textile company. Which one, Jay?"

"Prodesco," Jay said.

"Our father invented textiles for NASA," Dad said.

I'd heard about the curtains before, but not about the NASA inventions. That couldn't be true—if it were, why would my father have withheld that detail from stories about my grandfather? That's not just burying the lede; it's entombing it. I watched Jay to see if he'd look confused by Dad's bold, and maybe imagined, claim that my grandfather made space fabric, but my uncle nodded in confirmation.

"Anyway," Dad said, "our mother asked our father to have curtains made, and he thought she would want bright ones because she'd just made him paint all of the doors in the house a different color."

"I forgot about that!" Jay said.

"But Mom hated the curtains. She gave them to the neighbors. Whenever we went over there to play we'd say we were going to see the curtains. You know, your grandmother once made your grandfather put a waterfall in the living room?"

"A waterfall? How do you put a waterfall in a living room?"

"When you love somebody, you figure it out," Dad said. "Ha. Mom didn't like where Dad put the waterfall so she made him rip it out and do it again."

I looked at Jay, and he was still nodding along. It was comforting that he was confirming my father's stories, even if it was insanity like a waterfall in a living room. Maybe Dad meant a water *fountain*? Maybe this was Alzheimer's, revising history.

"You know," Dad continued, "we found the girl on Facebook."

"Susie," Jay said.

"Susie," Dad echoed. "She's all grown up now."

My father and uncle couldn't agree on which house was the curtains' house, and anyway, there weren't any ugly curtains in any windows. We got back in the car and drove a few minutes to Lenape Park, where there are some baseball fields and a trussed suspension bridge over a creek that was built as a public works project during the Great Depression. A sign at one end reads in red capital letters:

BRIDGE LIMIT
100 PEOPLE
NO
STOPPING
OR STANDING
ON BRIDGE
AT ANY TIME

Dad and Jay stopped in the middle and stood for another photo; my father flipped the bird while Jay gave him bunny ears. It was easy to imagine them scampering over this bridge sixty years ago, on their way to or from some kind of team practice. Somewhere I have a photo of little boy Ira in a baseball uniform. It's sparkling clean. Maybe that's why he took up the clarinet.

"One winter, when I was about twelve years old," Dad said, "the creek was frozen over and my mother warned us not to go on the ice because we'd fall in. So what did we do? Went on the ice. And fell in. Remember that, Jay?"

"I don't think so, I."

"Huh. Man, she was pissed. I remember we came home all wet and she wouldn't let us change clothes. Just sent us back to school."

"Are you sure, Dad?" I asked. "That's pretty messed up. You could have gotten sick."

"No," he said, looking confused, "I guess I'm not sure."

"It's okay, Dad," I said. "It was a long time ago."

"Was it?" he asked. "I guess it was."

I could see that Dad was fading and I was afraid he was going to start doing what Mom had warned me about, something called "sundowning." She said if he got too tired or overwhelmed toward the end of the day, he might start feeling anxious or scared, or start wandering around. She said it could get especially bad if he broke from his routine. Like, I don't know, taking a trip with two people he rarely sees, for example.

"Maybe we should call it a day and go eat something, Dad," I said. "Are you hungry?"

"Yeah."

We went for an early dinner at a pub near the Airbnb, and Dad raved over his beer, a seasonal pumpkin ale from Shock Top.

He drank only half but still wanted to go to the supermarket after dinner to buy a six-pack. I promised I would do it in the morning.

"We can't leave Perkasie without the beer, okay?" he said.

"You like it that much?"

"Mom will like it. We should bring her some."

"Mom doesn't drink beer."

"Okay, but I want to bring some home," he insisted.

"Okay, Dad."

What I didn't say, but wanted to, was that Shock Top is an Anheuser-Busch brand. We could probably buy it at any place in the country that sold beer. I could lie to Dad in the morning, promise that I bought some, then drive us all the way back to Massachusetts, stop for gas two minutes from his condo, and buy it at the gas station.

But this was Dad's trip. The whole point was to make him happy, and, so far, he was. I was worried that all of this nostalgia would be bad for his morale, that at some point it would hit him that this "vacation" was really a farewell tour.

"He knows that!" Mom said when I called to update her about our first day and shared my concern. "That's why this trip is such a wonderful gift. You're helping him say good-bye to the world on his own terms. It puts him back in control. And you know your father. He feels better when he's in control."

———

"Did we order yet?"

It was the fifth time my father had asked this question, over brunch at a restaurant that billed itself as "a fusion of flavors and cultural ideology." He was dipping the sleeve of his muck-colored field jacket into a ramekin of Creole aioli, and he had a shred of pulled pork in his beard. A few years ago, a few weeks ago, I would have rolled my eyes at his ridiculous Dad joke. *Very funny, Dad. YES, we ORDERED, ha ha.* But my father wasn't joking.

"Look down, Dad," I said, trying to stay calm but really, really feeling pushed to the limits of my patience. "Look down at your plate."

I didn't say "fucking plate," but everyone knew that's what I meant. Jay put his hand gently on Dad's arm.

"You've been enjoying your lunch, I," he said. "It's right there."

Dad blinked a few times and looked down. "Oh," he said, and you could smell the gears grinding as he remembered that we were halfway through a meal. He dipped a cold fry into ketchup and tried to be Joe Cool casual about taking a bite, but his hands were shaking. For nearly an hour he'd been taking birdlike nibbles of his food, whenever he remembered that he had food in front of him. Unlike me, our waitress was an angel of patience. Her name was Peaches.

Brunch was in historic New Hope, once a hub of American industry and now a tourist town on the banks of the Delaware River, about seven miles north of George Washington's legendary crossing and not far from Amish country.

"Save room for dessert?" Peaches asked when she came by to clear plates.

"No thanks," I said, at the same that time Dad said: "Dessert!" and gave her two thumbs-up.

"You remember the year I worked for Max Brenner?" he asked Jay.

"Who?" I asked.

"The chocolate company. There's one on Boylston Street."

Oh yeah. Max Brenner is a chain of dessert restaurants that describes itself as "a chocolate sensory immersion that encourages you to open your mind about how you connect with chocolate." I got a salted caramel hot chocolate there once, and it was the best sex I've ever had.

"You worked at the Boylston Street store?"

"No, not a store," Dad said. "Back when I was a kid your grandmother sent me out to California one summer to live with her sister, probably because I was a pain in the ass. I worked for a guy named Max Brenner. We called him the candy man. Nice guy. Hard worker. He made us work hard."

"What did you do for him?"

"Just helped him out. I remember a lot of vacuuming. Nice guy."

"But did you do anything with the chocolate?" I asked. "Was this before he started the restaurants? Did you help him start them?"

"We'd go to the beach on the weekends. This must have been near Bernice's place." Bernice was my grandmother's sister. "She had rusty old lawn chairs for us to take, and we set 'em up in the sand and watched people surfing. Max Brenner. The candy man. Did I ever tell you that I worked for him one summer?"

"Yes, Dad, you are literally telling me about it right now."

I liked hearing new stories from Dad's past, but it made me sad to think that I'd never know if they were true, if it was *Dad* talking, or the Alzheimer's, or some combination of the two. "Waterfall" vs. "water fountain." Although, I guess, it had been a long time since I'd trusted my father's version of the truth, anyway. I'd never been able to ask him about the books because I was afraid of the consequences of broaching a difficult subject. And I'd never be able to ask about things like rusty lawn chairs and candy men, because I didn't want to push my sad, sick Dad too far.

After brunch we went to pore over informational placards at Washington Crossing Historic Park, right where the icy Christmas battle magic happened. It's embarrassing but true that I didn't know much about it; only what I'd gleaned from Emanuel Leutze's famous painting *Washington Crossing the Delaware*. Nobody's messing around with fancy names or branding here. *Call it what it is! Why are we fucking around with this, guys?* "There is a fountain in this town." "Washington crossed here." "Here is a painting of him crossing."

I found it comforting. Except for "New Hope." I found that cruel.

After brunch, Dad wanted to walk along the stretch of the Delaware Canal that runs behind Main Street, but first: "Dunkin' Donuts!" he cried, pointing up the block. Sure enough, thar she blew.

Styrofoam cups in hand, we wandered down the dirt path next to the canal, past the Locktender's House, which was once just that and was now a small museum dedicated to just that. Sometimes Dad and Jay walked together, sometimes Dad charged ahead while I chatted with my uncle; got to know him, really. It's a little strange to be thrown into such an intense caretaking experience with someone you barely know, even if they are family. I guess it's also a little strange to barely know someone who's your family. But I liked Jay a lot, and it felt natural to talk openly with him. It reminded me of when I met Sam, and our shared hometown history immediately put me at ease.

My father posed for a photo next to a wooden fence the color of old blood. His glasses were too far down the bridge of his nose, his Indiana Jones fedora too floppy in his face. His head looked so small. It reminded me of little kids dressing up in their parents' clothes.

Some New Hope residents whose homes backed up to the canal had gone all out with gardening and decorating, so that trail walkers like us would have more to look at than water and trees. Dad quacked at some ducks and marveled at a homemade art installation: an androgynous mannequin with black eyeliner and plump shrimp lips. He/she/ze/they were wearing what looked like Israeli military fatigues, and casually gesturing to a pink birdhouse.

"Huh," Dad said.

Later, he posed for another photo in front of a gift shop on South Main Street called You the Man. Its old-timey sign featured an illustration of a king on a throne with a shield, for some reason. Maybe it's a famous illustration, or a famous king, and I was too ignorant to know, like how I didn't know that Washington crossed the Delaware with thousands of troops and horses, not just a boat or two, like in the painting. It does make sense that if anyone's going to be known as the man, it's a king. Can you imagine being the king, but nobody thinks you're the man? How embarrassing.

We went into a lot of weird little stores to pick up weird little things. Dad wanted to get something for the baby and chose a psychotic-looking puppy dog; it was blue and textured like stucco, with crinkly ears that sounded like those people you hate at the movie theater, who struggle to open their box of Milk Duds during a critical moment. On the way out I noticed a tin bathtub full of plastic baby dolls that would absolutely come alive and eat us later.

"Dunkin' Donuts?" Dad asked when we got outside, oblivious to the half-full coffee cup he was already holding.

"You wanted to poke around at some antiques shops," Jay reminded him, "to find something for Carolyn."

"Antiques!" Dad said, and we crossed the river into New Jersey where there were several antiques stores in one block. My father found a delicate enameled jewelry box for my mom, and some metal airplanes to hang in the baby's room that were undoubtedly covered in lead paint.

Dad fell asleep in the car on the way back to the Airbnb. When we arrived I shook him carefully awake, and as he came to, he made a sweet snargley sound.

"Hi, honey," he said, so sleepy. "Did we make it to the curtains?"

"We went yesterday, Dad," I said. "Want to take a nap and then go get dinner at the pub with the pumpkin beer?"

"Pumpkin beer," he said.

I helped him out of the car, then offered him my arm as we trudged up the stone porch steps. We stayed that way, arms linked, all the way up to the second floor. He kissed me on the cheek when we reached his bedroom.

"Will you wake me up for dinner?" he asked.

"Of course."

He kissed me on the cheek again and put a hand on my belly. "Bigfoot," he said, and laughed softly, like he couldn't believe it.

"Try to get some rest, Dad," I said, and ruffled his hair, so soft and thin.

"Okay. See you in the morning."

"Just a nap right now, Dad. It's only three o'clock."

"Okay. Then can we see the curtains?"

"They're not there anymore, remember?"

"Oh yeah," he said.

Dad kissed my cheek one more time and slipped into his room. I could hear the bed squeak, then the consecutive thuds of two tossed shoes hitting the floor. I stood in the hallway for a minute, listening, breathing, until the other side of the door was still. Then I went upstairs to my pull-out couch, pulled out my laptop, and googled Max Brenner's company history, to suss out what Dad might have spent a teenage summer doing for that nice-guy, hardworking candy man. The website said that the company was founded in 1996 by two Israeli guys, Max Fichtman and Oded Brenner, who just combined their names because they thought it sounded good. There was no actual "Max Brenner."

Then I tossed myself into the thick black hole of a good cry.

———

When it was over, Jay flew home to Wisconsin, Dad and I packed up the rental car with our suitcases and the leftover groceries, including two and a half boxes of Trader Joe's O's. Then we headed home. There were no Pennsylvania Turnpike questions or Dunkin' Donuts demands for several hours; we just listened to music and Dad told me stories. He was completely energized by our trip, and chattered happily about his childhood, and his high school jazz bands, and the time he spent backpacking through Europe with his college best friend. He talked a lot about my mom and told me the familiar story of how they met.

"She was beautiful," he told me, "and too smart to let some schmuck like me take her out. I had to get creative."

I let Dad talk for hours, partly because he was such a good storyteller, partly because I was in excruciating pain. I'd woken up with a dull ache in my gut that I'd thought was indigestion, but by the time we reached the New York border my entire left side felt cramped and stabby. It felt like I was being pinched by someone with claws, like a witch, or a wolverine. I didn't want to worry my dad, and I didn't want to stop, so I hunched over a little and drove until, somewhere in Westchester County, he spotted a Dunkin' Donuts and we pulled over. I had to kind of hobble inside, and Dad noticed.

"Bigfoot?" he asked, concerned.

"Yeah," I said, wincing, "I'm just feeling a little bit cramped."

"How about I drive?" he said. "You can stretch out in the back and have a little nap if you want to."

"You can't drive, Dad."

"Sure I can."

"You're not supposed to, remember?"

"Oh yeah."

I made it, somehow, even though by the time we hit the bridge alongside the little marina near my parents' place, the witch's pinch had moved further south, to my cervix.

Finally home at the honky-tonk condo, Mom was waiting with her hands clasped, excited to hear about our adventures. She gave my dad a big hug and a kiss while Callie jumped up on his leg. They were so happy to have him home. I watched as Mom tenderly led Dad over to the couch and handed him a mug full of tea that she'd already made for him.

I hobbled upstairs to call my doctor, who told me to get to the ER immediately.

When I told my parents, Dad was beside himself. He wanted to drive me. He didn't care that he wasn't supposed to. He was my dad, he kept saying, and dads take care of their kids. I gave him a hug and a kiss and pretended it wasn't a big deal, even though my doctor was worried that I was having a late miscarriage. By then I was twenty-four weeks pregnant. The baby had eyelashes now. He was the size of an ear of corn.

At the hospital they rushed me into a room with its own bathroom, and I tried to pee but it just felt like knives. A nurse hooked me up to a bunch of machines, and a doctor squirted me with goo and pressed an ultrasound probe to where the pain was the most intense. We could see That Guy on the monitor, tumbling around like a mermaid, healthy as a sea horse.

"False alarm," the doctor said. "Looks like you just had a cyst that ruptured. Look at this healthy little guy! Oops, sorry, you knew you were having a boy?"

"Yes," I said, and started to tear up.

"It's okay!" the doctor said, and she reached down to squeeze my hand. "He's okay. He's big!"

She wiped the goo off my stomach and printed out some pictures from the ultrasound.

"Here," she said, handing them to me, "add these to the family album."

I cried for the entire drive home, so relieved that That Guy was okay, and so relieved that I felt relieved.

When I got back to the honky-tonk condo, my dad was waiting in the living room with a cable-knit sweater vest and a cold mug of tea.

"He made the tea for you right after you left," Mom murmured in my ear. "He's been so worried."

My dad draped the sweater vest around my shoulders and handed me the tea.

"Is Bigfoot okay?" he asked.

"Yeah," I said. "False alarm."

"I wish you'd have let me drive," he said. "You could have stretched out in the backseat."

"It's okay, Daddy," I said. When was the last time I'd called him that? At least twenty years. He gave me a soft, sweet kiss on the crown of my head, and patted my shoulder.

I slurped the cold tea, and my mom fed me some dinner, and I told them about how happy and flippy the baby looked on the ultrasound monitor and gave them the pictures from the ER doctor. Mom propped them up on top of a dresser, among a cluster of framed family photos.

Later, upstairs, I locked myself in a bathroom to call Sam, to tell him the gist of the trip, and about the quick ER visit. There was no reason to do that. I had plenty of privacy in the guest bedroom. But, I don't know— When I was a kid, during thunderstorms I'd bring a blanket, a pillow, and a pile of books into the bathroom so I could hunker down in the (waterless) bathtub. It made me feel safe. I'm sure it upset anyone who needed to pee.

"He's going," I whispered, climbing into the tub and sliding down the wall until I was sitting, hugging my knees. "My dad. He's not the same. I don't think he'll ever be the same."

"I'm so sorry," Sam said. "That sounds so hard."

"I love him."

"I know."

"And That Guy," I said, starting to cry. "I was so scared. And I'm so glad I was scared."

"Me too."

"I think I love him."

"I know," Sam said.

I sniffed a little snorgle and wiped my nose on one of Mom's decorative washcloths. "You do?"

"Of course."

"I was afraid that I'd never love him."

"I wasn't," Sam said.

"You weren't?"

"I knew you'd love him. You're his mama."

"I'm scared for my dad," I said.

"I know."

"He's dying."

Sam was quiet for a second, then he cleared his throat and said: "I know."

Chapter 15

FIFTY-FIFTY

Something about that Perkasie trip unlocked a new stage of my dad's decline. Over the next few months he talked nonstop about the same childhood memories and half-baked adult ideas, over and over again. He wanted to move back to Bucks County; he wanted to reconnect with classmates and neighbors he hadn't seen in half a century. He wanted to go back to the pub with the pumpkin beer, even though my mom had started buying it for him every week at the supermarket. He'd take two swigs of the bottle and then forget all about it.

Dad wanted to do all of this moving and reconnecting and pumpkin-beering ASAP. "Before my condition takes over," he'd say. Never Alzheimer's or "the disease" or "this scary bullshit."

It was a lot.

But I mostly just had to listen to it. I didn't have to live it, like Mom did. She's the one who had to be there every day, restocking Dad's raisin bagels and reminding him how to trim his beard and nodding encouragingly at his relentless promises to get the business up and running so that once he was gone she'd be taken care of, but that he'd never felt better anyway. I didn't have to do any of that. I just had to stay on the phone for however long

I wanted to, and then I could say something about how work was really busy or the baby was really kicking so I'd have to go, and then I'd hang up and feel relieved that I didn't have to hear anything more about pumpkin beer, and then I'd feel ashamed of my own impatience.

Strangely, he'd stopped mentioning the sex books to me. I mean, thankfully. But they'd been a hot topic between us for so long. I didn't want to ask about them, in case it reminded him that, oh yeah, he needed to send his daughter more cartoons of humping clowns. Mom said that he was working furiously on a children's story about a camel named Humphrey.

"He also really needs you to write down those bedtime stories," she told me. "For the baby. He's so determined to pass them on, as his gift to you."

"I love that," I said. "What happened with, you know, the other books?"

"Just leave it alone," she said.

"Did you talk to him about them?"

"I didn't have to," she said. "He's figured out that nobody is interested in them, and he's still trying to get the business going. He thinks that children's books are the answer."

"You know there's no business, right?" I asked, and in hindsight, that was a cruel question.

"I know," Mom said sadly. "But he needs something to keep him going. He's really spiraling. It's happening faster than we thought it would."

As Dad's Alzheimer's progressed, so did my pregnancy. My belly swelled to the size of a small wrecking ball. My feet weren't too far behind. Sam and I bought a crib, hung light-blocking curtains in the baby's room, and made a list of names we both loved. Colin was the top choice for both of us. I can't remember why, to be honest. I wish I had a specific story, but I'm sure we just both came across Colin on an internet list of cool baby names, and liked the sound of it. We couldn't decide, though.

A coworker—who I suspected was the person who gave me *Ina May's Guide to Childbirth*—emailed me a link to a short documentary about orgasmic birth. A woman in labor floats serenely in an oversized kiddie pool, then her partner leans over to kiss her and she goes a little googly-eyed. I watched it in the A-hole and immediately deleted the email.

I wouldn't be having an orgasmic birth.

I'd be having a very clinical one.

Around Christmas 2014, we learned that I needed a C-section. That Guy had settled into a breech position, feet pointing down, head snuggled up near my ribs. Upside down. I was due in less than a month, and I'd started seeing a new OB, whom I'll call NOB.

NOB talked me through the dangers of trying to deliver a breech baby vaginally. Honestly, it was fine with me. There's a lot of hysteria on the internet about C-sections, but I liked the certainty of making an appointment to calmly stroll into a hospital and have a doctor remove That Guy from my body with surgical precision. Plus, come on. Who wants their vagina destroyed? And anyway, that orgasmic birth video seemed a little too theatrical to be real.

NOB gave me some options for trying to get him to turn around, which included cat/cow yoga poses (okay); an Eastern medicine technique that involved burning charcoal pencils next to my pinkie toes (…okay); and an external cephalic version, or ECV, wherein a small team of medical professionals tries to manually maneuver the baby into a head-down position. (Okay, no.) I know someone who had an ECV, and she said they put her in a long room, so narrow she could touch the walls on either side of her hospital bed as she lay there. She thought that maybe the room was so small because the hospital had tried to cram as many rooms into the building as possible, but then the medical team came in and took their positions on either side of her, bracing their feet against the walls for leverage as they dug their fingers into her belly and tried to scoop and cup the baby through my friend's skin, through the walls of her uterus.

"There's a fifty-fifty chance that an ECV will work," NOB told me and Sam, "so the odds are pretty good. I recommend we schedule you for one ASAP."

"Well," Sam said, "you mean the odds are equally good that it will work, and that it won't."

"What do you mean?" she asked.

"You said fifty-fifty," Sam said. "So it's just as likely that the ECV won't work as it is that it will work."

"Fifty percent likely that it will work," NOB said. "Those are good odds."

"They're equally bad odds," Sam said.

Going toe-to-toe with Sam about math or logic or just anything in general, really, can be exhausting. But I've known him long enough to understand that when he pushes back about probabilities, it's not because he's being pedantic, or insufferable. It's because he's feeling anxious or unnerved, and is seeking comfort in hard data.

"What happens if it doesn't work?" I asked NOB. "The baby just stays upside down?"

"That's one possibility," she said. "It could also be the case that the ECV is successful, but that the baby turns back around into a breech position. That's much less likely."

"What are the odds of that happening?" Sam asked.

"You don't have to answer that," I said quickly. "So that's it? It might work, it might not, it might work and then not?"

"Well…the other potential outcome is an emergency C-section," NOB said.

"When?" I asked.

"Right then and there," she admitted. "You could go into preterm labor, or the placenta could separate from the uterus, or a few other scenarios that would necessitate an immediate C-section."

I looked over at Sam and he was on his phone, no doubt frantically searching for data about the correlations between external cephalic versions and C-sections.

"That's it, then?" I asked. "Yoga, and/or smoke my feet, and/or play spin-the-baby, and/or hopefully not have an emergency C-section?"

"Of course," NOB said, "we could always just schedule you for a C-section and keep checking to see if the baby flips on his own."

"Great!" I said quickly, before Sam could google anything further. "Sign me up."

So that's what we did. We made an appointment to have a baby on January 12, 2015. Sam put it into our shared online calendar as "That Guy is born."

Chapter 16

THAT GUY IS BORN

That Guy did not flip on his own, so on January 12, we went to the hospital at 6:45 in the morning, as we'd been instructed. Also, per my pre-op instructions I hadn't eaten anything for twelve hours, and had scrubbed my entire body down with orange disinfectant surgical soap. I wonder why they make you do that so far in advance? So much time passes between the disinfecting and the surgery.

NOB herself didn't perform C-sections, so a different doctor would be doing the surgery. It was scheduled for nine o'clock, and I felt lucky that I wouldn't even go into labor, just lie around watching TV, bloated as a butterball turkey, until it was time to carve me up.

But nine o'clock came and went. There was a woman who needed an emergency C-section, so I got bumped. Then there was another emergency. Then two more.

Normally this wouldn't have thrown things so out of whack, but the hospital had just finished building a brand-new facility in a different part of town, and they were in the process of moving their entire birth center. I was in their "old" location, and the whole wing was pared down to basics: only one operating room

was operating; only a few recovery rooms were occupied. The
nurses plotted their new commutes in hushed tones, thrilled by
their improving parking situations and lunch options. The dust
bunnies clumped at the foot of my IV stand looked like even *they*
couldn't wait to hop on out of there. Hearing the place where
someone's going to stick you with knives described as "old"
doesn't inspire a ton of confidence.

By two o'clock they still weren't ready for me. I hadn't eaten in
nineteen hours, which to a pregnant woman feels more like the
time it takes to read *The Master and Margarita*, in that you can't
really quantify it, just endure it, confused and furious.

Sam decided he was starving so he went to a Subway across
the street and brought back a foot-long Italian that seemed to
me, a greedy and frantic buffalo person, more like fifteen feet. I
wasn't supposed to eat before the surgery just in case something
went wrong, but I begged for a bite anyway. Just one.

"I'm sorry, baby!" Sam said, wide-eyed and sincere, through a
delectable mouthful of cheese and meat.

"I don't want to miss anything!" he said. "I was going to eat
this at Subway, but what if they called you in and I wasn't back
yet? I'm sorry! Look, here—" He turned his back on me to face
the window. "I'll eat like this!"

And he did. I could hear it. Every smacky little mouth chomp.

If I hadn't been so hangry, I would have laughed at the similar-
ities between this and my own birth, when Dad ate a hamburger
with his back turned on Mom. I can't remember if I ever told
Sam that story, or if this was just a cruel coincidence.

When a nurse came in to let me know that, sorry, there was
another emergency and they probably wouldn't be ready for me
until around four, I asked her if I should just go home.

"You can certainly go if that's what you want to do," she said.

"But we'd have to formally discharge you, then when you come back we'd readmit you, and put your IV back in, and you might go back on the waiting list if there's another emergency."

"You don't want to go home, babe," Sam said. "It'll be your turn soon. I know it feels like forever because you haven't eaten anything—"

My stomach made a beastly noise and the baby kicked me in the cervix, just once. Just to make a point.

"—but we're so close and don't you think you'll regret it if we leave? It's okay. I promise I won't eat in here again."

The nurse raised an eyebrow. "You ate in here? In front of her?" she asked.

"Right?!" I said.

"I'm *sorry*," Sam said again, brushing a crumb from his cheek.

Finally, finally, around 4:30, another nurse appeared. I wish I could remember anyone's name. All I remember are faceless women in pink hospital scrubs.

"Your turn!" she said. "Ready to have a baby?"

Holy shit, I thought. I'd spent the entire day feeling like this was dragging on, but now it all felt like it was happening too fast. "What about Sam?"

"You stay here for a few minutes," she said to Sam. "I'll be back with your OR scrubs."

"Oh, I get scrubs, babe!" Sam said. "It's just like I'm a doctor on a medical procedural television program!" He said "program" like *pro'grum*, which was one of our million secret language in-jokes that we'd amassed over the years, like private little treasures.

"Ready?" the nurse asked, even though it didn't matter.

"I love you," I whispered to Sam.

"I love you too," he whispered back. "Let's go meet That Guy."

The faceless nurse (sorry, whoever you are!) led me down the hall to the operating room. I had to roll my IV cart along and was grateful to have something to cling to.

The OR looked like an alien abduction must feel, with huge, round lamps hovering like curious bystanders over a stainless steel slab. Everything smelled like unflavored mouthwash.

"Can you curl over into a C?" the nurse asked as several people in several shades of scrubs appeared. It was epidural time. "Take some deep breaths and then try to hold still. Do you want me to hold your hands?" She didn't wait for an answer, just took them and gave them a squeeze. It was kind of nice.

"Where's Sam?" I asked and tried to focus on holding still instead of panicking. I think they purposely make you curl over before the anesthesiologist comes into view so you don't see their arsenal of needles.

"He'll be here soon," the nurse said. I really should give her a name. "We usually try to have significant others wait until the epidural is in before we have them come in."

"Why?"

"You know? I don't actually know," she said, and then drew a blue paper sheet up over my face.

"Hey babe!" I heard Sam call. "Look at me!" He emerged from behind the sheet in a collared paper jacket and shower cap and did a cute little hoedown dance. "Look, I brought my phone so I can take pictures of your guts."

The actual doctor appeared—the attending OB who would be performing the surgery. I'll call her Dr. N-NOB, for "doctor not NOB." This is all ridiculous.

"Sir, we actually recommend that you don't look over the blue sheet," N-NOB said.

A man appeared and introduced himself as Peter, the anesthesiologist. "Hello, Ms. Alterman!" he said. "Congratulations, you're about to meet your baby! I'm going to put some pressure on your abdomen, and all you need to do is tell me if it hurts."

Beyond the blue curtain I could feel a mild push against my belly, like someone was teasing it with the eraser end of a pencil.

"I can feel it."

"Does it hurt?"

"No, it's just annoying."

"Good," Peter said, and he pulled the curtain down and showed me what was surely a late nineteenth-century lobotomy instrument, or a fondue fork for giants. "I was poking you with this. See how sharp it is? Enough to break the skin."

"That's the point, right?" I joked weakly. "Get it? 'Point.' Like, it's supposed to break my skin so you can get the baby out but also, it's pointy."

"Funny," Peter said, without laughing. He disappeared behind the curtain.

"I thought it was funny," I said to myself.

"Me too, baby," Sam said loyally, squeezing my hand.

"How am I doing?" I asked.

"I don't know," he said. "How are you doing?"

"No, you're supposed to tell me how amazing I am," I whined. "I know all of these men who post on Facebook about how their wives were beautiful warriors when they gave birth."

"Do you want me to post something on Facebook?"

Before I could whine some more at Sam about how he should be calling me a beautiful warrior, I heard someone call out, "Here he comes!" and Sam let go of my hand to pop up over the paper sheet, like a curious meerkat. A meerkat with an iPhone.

"I see all your guts, baby!" he said, and started taking phone pictures. "Wow, so many guts."

I felt a huge tug somewhere below the belt, then heard a single, tiny squawk of protest.

"Is that him?" I asked. "Already? That was so fast!"

"Getting him out doesn't take very long," Dr. N-NOB called out from behind the curtain. This whole curtain thing made me think of *The Wizard of Oz*. The great and powerful N-NOB. "The majority of the procedure is putting you back together."

"Oh," I said, then: "Wait. Why isn't he crying?"

Dr. N-NOB didn't answer. Nobody did. I could hear a flurry of activity, like the bleeps and bloops of machines, and the general sounds of hospital goings-on. All I saw was blue sheet, six inches from my face.

"Why isn't he crying?" I asked again. Sam left to go investigate.

I tried to calm myself down by taking some deep breaths and thinking about my own birth, and how I'd also come out of my mother with just a squawk.

In an instant, Sam was back by my side. "Hi, babe!" he said, with a smile that was all winner winner chicken dinner. He held out his phone. "I took some pictures so you can see That Guy! He's real little. Look at his little frog legs!"

I heaved a sigh of relief. At least, I think I did. I couldn't really feel any part of my body except for my face and arms. But I saw my chest rise and fall, so I'm assuming.

"I don't want to just see a picture of his little frog legs," I said, "I want to touch his little frog legs."

Dr. N-NOB finally showed her surgical-masked face.

"Hi, Ms. Alterman," she said. "The baby looks good, but we want to take him down to the NICU for a bit, to make sure his lungs are clear and he's getting enough oxygen."

"The what?"

"The NICU." She said it like "nick you." "The neonatal intensive care unit."

Oh no. "Is he breathing?"

"Yes!" she said. "Don't worry. We do this a lot with C-section babies."

"Can I hold him? Before you take him?"

"Absolutely!" she said, and disappeared behind the curtain again.

And then, there That Guy was.

I can't remember who, but someone slipped a squirmy, purple person onto my chest, then covered us with a warm blanket. A nurse helped me untangle a few tentacles of IV tubes so I could fully fold my arms around the baby. My little baby boy. My son.

I couldn't see anything but the crown of a hospital-issue stocking cap, but when the baby's skin touched mine I felt some kind of energy move between us—strange, because I still couldn't feel my own chest. Just a warm swell. It reminded me of when you make a grilled cheese sandwich, and there's that Rubicon moment when the cheese melds with the bread and you can't fully separate them anymore.

Man, I was hungry.

"Hi, little guy," I murmured. "I'm your mama. You found me."

As soon as I said it, my heart cracked wide open. I couldn't believe how much I already loved this sweet creature.

"You found me," I said again, but through a throat choked with relief it sounded more like *goo fow nee.* "Goo fow nee."

He squawked another baby bird sound. We lay like that for a few minutes, him squawking, me crying, Dr. N-NOB stuffing offal back into my body. I pictured her cramming intestines into my open cavity the same way you fight to fit a squishy pillow into a pillowcase.

Sam gently kissed my forehead. "They need to take him now, babe," he said softly. "Do you want me to stay here with you?"

"No. Go with him," I said, rubbing my son's soft and sweet back. "Go with him."

He took our baby gently and then, it was just me on a table.

"Doing okay?" Peter asked.

"Yeah," I said.

"Can you feel anything?"

"Just some tugging. And...ow."

"Ow?" he asked. "There shouldn't be an 'ow.' Hold on, let me crank up the juice." A soft, warm flush spread up my IV arm, and it set me adrift.

"What did you do?" I asked.

"Increased the intensity of the anesthesia, and gave you a mild sedative," he said. "You shouldn't feel any pain now."

"Bless you," I said.

"What are you going to name your son?" Peter asked.

"Colin," I said.

"Great name," said Dr. Nameless. "Why Colin?"

"We just...like...it," I said, and my own voice sounded like a foghorn in the growing distance from consciousness.

———

I awoke to the sounds and sensations of my own exorcism.

"Huh-wahuhhhhhhhhhnnngg."

That's the best I can do to capture the sound of my vomiting. *"Huh-wahuhhhhhhhhhnnngg.* Oh god. Ow! Fucking ow. *Huh-wahuhhhhhhhhhnnngg."*

Everything was hazy, but through the haze was insane pain. I was lying on my back, propped up at 45 degrees, and everything—

my throat, my face, the gash in my lower abdomen—groaned in protest whenever I heaved. *I'm going to rip a stitch*, I thought. *How many stitches do I have? Or do I have staples? Do staples rip?* "*Huh-wahuhhhhhhhhnnngg.*"

"Hi, babe!" Sam materialized by my side, casually holding a pink plastic bedpan. I grabbed it from him and got sick again.

Another faceless nurse appeared and handed me a small waxed-paper cup full of sweet-smelling red liquid. It reminded me of the bug juice we slurped at summer camp; that nasty neon sugar water in a bottomless Igloo cooler.

"You're just having a reaction to the anesthesia," she said. "Vomiting is totally normal; it should be over very soon. Try to take some fluids if you can."

I drank the juice. It ended up in the bedpan. I drank more. Same. When my abs contracted it was torture from the inside out.

"Where's That Guy?" I moaned, groggy and froggy.

Sam smiled. "Oh, you mean That Guy Colin?" He pointed to a bassinet on wheels that reminded me of the pushcarts at small grocery stores, the ones that are just a steel skeleton with space to drop a basket in. Colin was in there, burritoed in a blanket. "Sleeping," Sam said. "The nurse says after a C-section, you're supposed to try to stand up and walk a little."

"Walk where?"

"Do you want to walk to the sink and brush your teeth?"

"Do I need to brush my teeth?"

Sam broke into a wide and teasing smile. "I don't know!" he said in the singsong voice he uses whenever he *does* know.

As soon as I could manage to talk without puking, we called our parents to tell them they had a Colin now. My mom cried the happiest tears. Dad kept saying, "Ha! Ha!" and, of course, signed off from our conversation with "Never wake a sleeping baby!"

I spent the next few days propped up in a hospital bed, sniffing Colin's head as he lay on my bare chest and thinking of smells it smelled even better than: like freshly baked bread, or sizzling bacon, or cinnamon rolls. It was mostly food smells, to be honest. Hospital food leaves a lot to be desired.

Sam and I took turns feeding and changing and singing to and staring at Colin. Every once in a while someone would show up to check my catheter or give me pain meds or knead my belly. They sent in a social worker, a chaplain, a photographer. Some excellent friends brought us sushi and booze.

When we finally went home, it was more of the same. Feed, change, sing, stare. We gave Colin little sponge baths and gently dabbed him dry with a yellow hooded towel that I think was supposed to make him look like a duck, but instead made him look like a duck was trying to eat him from the crown down.

Colin slept for only an hour or two at a time. Pretty normal for a baby, I guess, but I thought it would be easy to pop a bottle into his mouth and then pop him back into his crib and toss myself back into a chasm of deep sleep. Instead, I dozed on the brink of unconsciousness, never fully able to surrender, listening for tiny coughs or chokes or maybe even ghosts. I don't believe in spooky-ooky things, generally, but our house's history haunted me. Right after we moved in, a neighbor told us that in the 1940s, our house was home to a man named August DeMont. He was thirty-seven years old, an elevator mechanic, a father. One morning, he told his wife he was taking their five-year-old daughter, Marilyn, with him on an errand. He drove to the Golden Gate Bridge and convinced Marilyn to climb a railing, then jump hundreds of feet down into the Bay. Then he followed. He left a note in his car that said: "I and my daughter have committed suicide."

The story had made me feel sick when I first heard it. And now, it practically consumed me. Sometimes when I went in to feed Colin in the middle of the night, I'd linger in the rocking chair after he'd already fallen asleep in my arms, and I'd stare down at his sweet little face, and think about the DeMont family, wondering where Marilyn had slept and if August had ever sat up with her when she was sick or scared. I'd think about her poor mother, and how excruciating it must be to outlive your child, and I wondered if any of their ghosts were watching us.

Chapter 17

NEVER WAKE A SLEEPING BABY

A few weeks after we brought Colin home from the hospital, my parents flew out to visit. When they got to our house, Mom immediately wrapped Colin in a hug and nuzzled him close, and he tried to wrap his lips around her nose.

"Oop!" she laughed. "Babies always go for the nose. The nose knows!" she cooed at Colin. "Doesn't it, honey? What a sweet boy, my grandbaby boy! Grans and Pop love you so much!"

"What do you think, Pop?" I asked my dad, wrapping my arms around him for a hug. He was wearing a brown knit sweater vest, and beneath that a flannel shirt, and beneath that a T-shirt, and beneath that he felt like paper skin and crispy bones.

"Never wake a sleeping baby," he said.

"Okay. But what do you think about having a grandson?"

"I have a grandson!" he said. "It's wonderful. Don't you think it's wonderful?"

"I do," I said. "But you know, it's also really scary."

"We're constantly freaked out," Sam explained to my parents. "Like, if Colin makes a funny noise in his sleep, we're convinced that something is horribly wrong."

"Oh, well, that's normal," Mom said.

"Is it?" Dad asked her, and then asked me: "Is something wrong with the baby?"

"No, Dad," I said, "nothing's wrong."

"Everything is new," Mom said. "I used to stare at you for hours when you slept, just watching you breathe."

"I've been doing that too," I said. "I'm just, I don't know, I'm scared. I'm scared that he'll get sick or hurt and I won't know what to do about it. And then, it's so dumb, but this house is so old, and when I sit up with Colin at night I just get carried away thinking about scary things, even stupid scary things, and then I don't want to leave him alone."

My dad put one hand on my shoulder and looked me right in the eyes. "Did you know that when you were a baby, your mother took a dog bite for you?"

"What?" Sam asked. "Jeez."

"A German shepherd," Mom agreed. "I was walking you in the stroller and it came right up to us. It was going for you, but I jumped in the way. Took a chunk right out of my leg."

"She jumped right between you," Dad said. "Didn't stop to think about it, just did it."

"It could have killed you," Mom said. "It was going right for the stroller."

"She didn't think twice," Dad said. "Neither will you. Moms are always the scariest thing in the room."

"I hope so," I said. "Hey Dad, remember that little white gorilla you gave me?"

"Fergus!" he said. "Fergus the Dream Gorilla."

"His name was Fergus?" I said. "Are you sure? I don't remember him having a name."

"Fergus the Dream Gorilla," Dad said again. "He scared away the bad guys so you could sleep."

"Yeah," I said. "I've been thinking about him a lot. I wish I had someone to scare away the bad guys again."

"Nah," Dad said. "You're the gorilla now."

—————

My parents' visit was as painful as it was joyful. Sam went back to work so it was just the three of us, and after he left each morning I'd stare down the clock, counting the minutes until it was a reasonable hour to take Colin to my parents. We'd booked them an Airbnb several blocks away, so everyone could have as much sleep and space as possible. San Francisco being San Francisco, it was a fifteen-minute walk downhill from our place to theirs, and twice that in reverse. Dad was still measuring his daily exercise in ups and downs, but the up-up-up to our place was too much for him, so the very instant it hit 7:30 I'd load Colin in the stroller and walk him down-down-down to my parents. Then walk myself up-up-up and go back to bed for a few hours.

My father was so happy to grandparent, but also so pre-occupied. It was snowing back in Massachusetts and he asked about the weather constantly—he was worried about icy road conditions. He was worried that there'd be a snowstorm and the flight would be delayed, or diverted.

"But why do the roads in Massachusetts matter? You're here," I kept trying to point out, and Dad would get annoyed with me and say, "But when we get back. The roads could be bad."

Dad also obsessed over how they would get to the airport when it was time to go home. We talked about it multiple times a day, every day of their visit. I didn't understand what the big deal was—I'd picked them up at the airport; I could take them there again. Or, I could just put them in a taxi. This should have been a nonissue. But Dad brought this up again and again. He thought it would put me out to have to drive them, but he also insisted that taxis were sketchy and unreliable.

The shitty thing about Alzheimer's, besides all of the other shitty things about Alzheimer's, is that people who suffer from it are trying to make sense of the world around them all the time.

Dad constantly repeated the same questions with the same urgency because he felt lost and disoriented, and he couldn't remember that his questions had already been asked and answered. It was impossible to quell his anxiety, and it was just so exhausting. I wish I were a more saintly person, who never got annoyed with my vulnerable, unsettled father, but the truth is, I was constantly on the verge of screaming. I tried to be patient and truthful with him, because if I showed even a flicker of annoyance, it wounded him. He couldn't understand why his question had offended me, because he couldn't remember that he'd already asked it six times. My father's main concerns had narrowed, and were now all but limited to: the Pennsylvania Turnpike, Dunkin' Donuts, getting to the airport, getting home, and never waking a sleeping baby.

My mom told me that he couldn't sleep, and would pace the Airbnb all night muttering about snow. Once, he even tried to walk out the door at two in the morning, presumably to get a head start on foot for the pilgrimage to the airport.

They took a rest day so Dad could nap and do crossword puzzles, and Mom could keep an eye on him to make sure he didn't try to leave the apartment. As he slept, she made us massive batches of marinara and meatballs and chicken cacciatore. Bizarrely, they refused to do laundry at our house—Mom said it was so they didn't burden the new parents.

"That's ridiculous," I argued. "How is you using the washing machine a burden? It won't affect me in any way."

She ignored me and bagged up their laundry in a garbage bag to haul to a Laundromat in the neighborhood. Later that afternoon, she called and said, "Good news! I've found a solution to our problem!"

"What problem?" I asked, confused.

"Getting to the airport."

"Mom!" I growled, and Colin, asleep on my chest, gave a little sigh. "Jesus Christ. How many times do I need to tell you that this isn't a problem? I can just drive you."

She ignored me and explained that she'd "made friends with" a woman who very kindly offered to send her brother to drive my parents to the airport for just $80.

"I met her down in the village!" Mom trilled. "She's from Hawai'i!" She pronounced it huh-WAH-ee, with an enthusiastic pause between "WAH" and "ee."

"What *village*, Mom?"

"Your little village!"

I pinched the skin on the bridge of my nose, hard, and took a huge breath.

"Mom. I do not live in a 'village.' I live in a major city."

"It's such a sweet little street."

She was talking about 24th Street, the main drag of our San Francisco neighborhood, Noe Valley. There's a cheese shop there, and three toy stores, a bakery, several bars and restaurants, a few real estate agencies, one teeny store that sells only adult-sized footie pajamas, and the shell of a burned-down RadioShack.

"Not a village, Mom. And why do you trust a stranger over your own daughter?" I asked. This whole crisis over airport transportation was bonkers. This was supposed to have been a happy visit to meet a new baby and help a new mom. Instead, I was in a tizzy every day over my parents' panic about a simple drive.

"But you want us to take a taxi—those are driven by strangers. What's the difference?" she said, and she sounded indignant. Which was totally unfair. I was the one who had the right to feel indignant. "And anyway," she continued, "he's only going to charge us $80. It's a great price."

"That's extortion!" I said. "It's a twelve-minute drive to the airport! It should cost you $40, including tip! It should cost you nothing because *I said I would drive you myself!* You're telling me that you want to give $80 to a random stranger to drive you somewhere, but that a taxi is sketchy? What is wrong with you?"

"I can handle this myself," she sniffed. "Just leave it alone." And then she hung up.

I couldn't see at the time that my mom must not have been seeing things clearly, that she was as freaked out and tired as I was. But the source of my fatigue and fear was a happy one: a bouncy new baby. Mom's was an unraveling husband. I should have been kind about it, but I wasn't.

It stung, that all my parents seemed to focus on throughout the course of their visit was how it was going to end. But I didn't say anything. What was the point?

The day before they left I caught my dad sitting in our uncomfortable armchair, gently swaying, trancelike, as Colin napped in his arms. I snapped a quick phone picture, and the lighting is terrible. Colin looks yellow, and he is swimming in a pair of striped pajamas that won't fit for another few months. His tiny hand is gently clutching a fold of Dad's knit sweater. Neither of them is smiling. Both of them have their eyes closed.

It's the only photo I have of my father holding my son, and it's beautiful.

The camera flash caught Dad's attention, and his eyes fluttered open and he smiled, first at me and then down at Colin.

"Never wake a sleeping baby," he said, and closed his eyes again.

———

My parents did not get a ride to the airport from the Hawaiian woman's brother. They still refused to come with me, for reasons I will never understand or even hear come out of their mouths. I finally, miraculously, convinced them to let me send them to the airport in an Uber, though in order to convince them, I lied and said it was a car service that Sam sometimes used for work. We sprang for Uber's "black car" service, where a professional driver shows up in a sleek luxury SUV. And son of a fucking goat, it cost me $80.

My parents did not have any weather-related flight problems; they did not encounter icy roads on the drive home to the honky-tonk condo. They just went home, and we all just went on.

Chapter 18

SKILLED CARE

After my parents left, Sam's parents came, and left. And then it was just me and That Guy Colin for the rest of my maternity leave.

Those first few months felt like one long day. Feed, diaper, bathe, repeat. I watched Colin sleep—even in the middle of the night—just to make sure he kept breathing. Sometimes I'd reach up to take off my smudgy glasses so I could clean them, but—ow, fuck!—I'd poke myself in the eye. Because I wasn't wearing smudgy glasses. Those were just my smudgy eyes.

Parenting brought new, strange realities to my life that none of the baby books anticipated. I thought I'd already known, for example, what all of the human body fluids are.

Thankfully Colin didn't cry too much, but he didn't eat too much or sleep too much, either, or smile at all. Every time I brought him out in public some well-intentioned fire monster would say something like, "Aw, it gets better soon!" or "You're doing great, mama!" There was one man (of course) who passed by as I was struggling to maneuver the stroller into a café while I held the door open with my butt. "Wow," he said, "you've got your hands full!" And then he just kept walking.

The slog of childcare and housework was more bearable if I sang along to happy music, especially songs from Disney movies I'd loved as a kid. You haven't washed a stack of dishes, scrubbed down a shower, or rolled teeny little socks into tiny little balls until you've done those things while Broadway-belting a Disney song that suits the moment. I'm talking "Be Our Guest" from *Beauty and the Beast*, I'm talking "Spoonful of Sugar" from *Mary Poppins*, I'm definitely talking that gibberish "rubbity scrubbity" song from *The Sword in the Stone*. That's the Disney version of the legend of King Arthur, and it was one of Dad's favorites. I've never met a single other person who's seen or even heard of it.

I imagined myself as a lithe maiden, or a gracefully fluttering laundry fairy who sprinkled joy and clean undies around the apartment. In reality, I looked like a drunk ogre who'd fallen into a bag of clothes at a yard sale.

Colin loved all of it. The first time he smiled was when I swung him around in the air, listening to music from *The Lion King*. Babies are such stone-faced little sourpusses. All I'd wanted was a sign from that kid, That Guy, to show me that I was doing this whole blerging parenting thing correctly. That first smile was the best, best thing. My days went from feed, diaper, bathe, repeat, to creating opportunities for connecting with my son.

After that, every day we'd spend at least an hour singing and dancing together. Colin would smile his perky and porky little grin—sometimes he'd even laugh a little. I loved sharing my favorite music with my sweet baby. I wondered if that's how my parents felt when we were all bopping around in the living room together, listening to records.

In the midst of an afternoon diaper change, my playlist landed on "Part of Your World," from *The Little Mermaid*, and I immediately lifted Colin into the air for a dance. It's a song about wanting more than your life has to offer you, and for that I've always found it a little depressing. Relatable, too. But it's an uplifting song, and so hopeful. If you're not familiar, there's a turning point in the middle where the music crescendos and the mermaid, Ariel, has a moment of self-affirmation. She's tired of her soggy underwater existence and is ready to join a sisterhood of "bright young women, sick of swimming, ready to stand," and "stand" lasts for two full bars, like, "staaaaaaaaaand."

The music swells, and fuck yes, this is Ariel's moment of empowerment. And as I danced with my pantsless baby the music swelled, and *fuck yes*, this was my moment of empowerment. Motherhood. I was doing it. I was killing it. I raised my son high into the air like a lion cub destined to rule the pride (Disney, at this point I'd be happy to talk about a payment plan for sponsored content) and held that "staaaaaaaaaand" out for seven full counts, just like Ariel, and on the eighth beat, when I was really feeling myself, Colin peed into my mouth.

On the other side of the country, Mom and Dad were enjoying their own buffet of new and unpredictable struggles. For example, the day they discovered that my father had forgotten how to button his pants.

It happened during an Alzheimer's fund-raising walk, of course. My parents had formed a team with some friends from their local senior center and trained for the gentle two-mile route by walking extra ups and downs with Callie.

"Dad was so determined," Mom told me on the phone, and, thankfully, she was laughing.

Their team had barely begun to march from the starting line when, *whoosh*, Dad's pants hit his ankles like a magician's curtain drop.

"He had no idea what to do," my mom said with a chuckle. "I mean, we were walking along Route 1, with all of these cars whizzing by, and nobody could get his pants back up. And people felt sorry for us, but we just started laughing and couldn't stop. Don't feel bad; Dad was laughing too. It's good for us to have something to laugh about."

Mom also thought it was funny the night she woke up to find Dad looming over her, peering down in awe like she was a sleeping princess, or an award-winning calzone.

"I just want to kiss you," he told her, then leaned down to give her a peck and went back to sleep.

But it was a different kind of funny—not something that makes you laugh. Something that makes you suspicious.

Although the Alzheimer's had center stage, my dad had other, smaller health problems that caused him trouble. (They were un-related to the dementia, just products of being an aging man with a history of digestive tract problems. I'll allow him the dignity of keeping those details to a minimum.) He'd needed to have a few kidney stones broken up; he'd needed to have his gallbladder surgically removed. These are minor outpatient procedures, but they're painful, and stressful. Surgery and anesthesia can be extra stressful and confusing for dementia patients, but Dad seemed to have handled them just fine.

That's why nobody thought it would be a big deal when he needed another minor surgery, for some benign prostate situation that Mom said was causing all of his stones. And it wasn't a big deal at the time. It went well. The hospital sent him home with a bottle of pain meds and a temporary catheter to make the nights easier. Everyone felt great great great about it.

That first night home after the surgery, though, my dad woke up in the middle of the night, saw the catheter tube, and yanked it out of his own bladder in an absolute panic. He'd forgotten that it was supposed to be there, forgotten that it was a medical device and not, say, an alien invasion. He'd forgotten that he'd had surgery.

Mom spent the entire night trying to soothe him, and first thing in the morning, she took him back to the hospital, where they replaced the catheter and sent him home. That night, it happened again. Mom took him back. They replaced the catheter again, and sent him home again. He ripped it out *again*.

Mom put herself on 24/7 catheter watch, keeping the same intense eye on my dad that I kept on my son, watching his chest heave, listening for the cadence of his breath. My parents were on Medicare. Hiring in-home care wasn't an affordable option, and Mom didn't want to ask me to fly out and help. She kept all of this a secret from me.

Finally, she begged the hospital for support. They couldn't keep Dad, wouldn't, because there was no medical reason to do it. Instead, they referred him to an inpatient medical rehab center, so nurses could keep an eye on his catheter round the clock, and my mother could get some rest.

"As long as he needs skilled care," she told me, "then Medicare will cover his stay for one hundred days. After that, we're going to need to figure something out."

"Well what's 'skilled care'?" I asked.

"Medical needs," she said. "He's got the catheter, so that counts. Then, if he needs an IV for anything, or physical rehab."

"But what about, like, if he wakes up in the middle of the night and tries to leave the house again? Or turns on the burner and fills the house with gas?"

Mom was quiet for a second. "That doesn't count," she said.

Putting my dad in the rehab center made everything so much

worse, so quickly. He was still waking up confused every night, only now, he was in a strange bed in a strange room, no familiar faces in sight, just a weird old roommate, Al, who Mom said spent his days watching weird old TV shows in a weird old armchair. They roomed an *Alzheimer's* patient with a guy named *Al*. Believe me, if Dad had been in the mood for irony, that one would have set him rolling on the floor. He still had a catheter, was still ripping it out and having it replaced all the time. My mom visited every day, and he'd beg her to please, please take him home. She'd call to update me from his room, and he'd grab the phone from her hand and beg me to please beg my mom to take him home.

The hardest call to take was the day he burst into silent tears. I thought he'd just paused midconversation for a drink of water or something, but then I heard a sniff, and in a tiny voice he said, "I just want to be with my family. I don't want to be here. I'm going to die here." He sounded like a lost little boy, looking for his mother.

"Oh, Dad," I said, and my heart was a shattered glass bowl. "It's okay. You're not going to die! You just need to stay a little longer so you can get better, and then Mom's going to take you—"

I heard a rustle, then a sharp thud, then the line went dead. Mom told me later that he'd thrown the phone against the wall and broken it.

Mom took Dad out of the center whenever he was feeling up to it. They took Callie for short, slow walks, or went for lunch at Haley's Ice Cream, a fabulous retro joint with checkered floors and teal booths and a weird little carved-wood fisherman who kept watch out front by the trash cans. Dad liked to order hot fudge sundaes, cheeseburgers, or giant cups of coffee ice cream swirled with orange sherbet. He could handle only a few bites at a time, but he savored them and made weird, annoying mouth noises about the "extraordinary flavors." Mom would coo, "That's good, huh, I? Mmm. Good! Yum!" while high school athletes hanging out after practice eavesdropped and laughed. Who could blame them for laughing at two old people making orgasm sounds about extraordinary flavors?

I left Colin home with Sam and flew to Massachusetts to visit my dad in the rehab center. I wanted to just be back there, to move there, or to take Colin for an extended stay. It would have been impossible, I think, without quitting my job, and we couldn't afford that. San Francisco rents are criminally expensive, plus, all of these cross-country flights were bleeding us dry. I didn't love the work I was doing, but it wasn't torture, just tedious. My company was incredibly understanding about all of these trips. They let me work remotely so that I didn't blow through my vacation time, and they left me alone while I was gone, as long as I turned my work in on time and called in for meetings. I mentally seesawed between deeply resenting arguments about adding "now" to the end of "Check out our new Texas Red Dirt country music station," and feeling deeply grateful for the distraction.

Mom took me for my first visit to the rehab center, a low, wide brick building with a massive New Orleans–style porch that had stately white pillars and two verandas. Like someone took a suburban apartment complex and tried to make it seem grand. Across the street from Hope Community Church. Come on.

I was nervous, but I couldn't decide if I was scared to see my dad or just scared to see how we were forcing him to live. What if he started crying when he saw me, or shouting? What if he hated me for not breaking him out of here? What if he had zero reaction to me at all, because he didn't know me?

Inside, Mom and I signed in and were buzzed through a security door, then passed by a community room where a few of the residents were watching TV and having gentle conversations about grandchildren. Several of the staff greeted my mother warmly.

"Don't be alarmed," she warned me as we headed toward Dad's room. "He looks very skinny and he's been getting more easily confused. But it's still him, okay? It's important for you to remember that."

My father's room was a short walk down a long hallway and reminded me of the hospital room I'd stayed in after my C-section. Dad was waiting for me, perched delicately on the edge of a chair. He looked more frail than I'd expected, like a scraggy little bird after a hard winter. He smiled, though, and stood up to give me a long, warm hug.

The room was bigger than I'd expected, but with few frills and almost zero privacy. His bed was just inside the door, along the left wall, and he had a little nightstand where Mom had set his CD player. There was a thin cotton curtain between him and Al, who was indeed in a weird armchair watching weird TV. They shared a bathroom. I asked Dad what he thought about that, and he just made a pained face, gave two thumbs-down, and shook his head. Still him, all right.

Dad said he was feeling great, so Mom and I took him out for a slow stroll on the Clipper City Rail Trail, a serene corridor that's lined with gardens, granite walls, and works by local artists. My favorite is a massive sculpture of two soaring sparrows, touching wings. I snapped a photo of my parents in front of a steel-and-wood sculpture of a horse named Clyde. Mom's hair looks extra bouncy, and Dad is hunched over a walker, all salt-and-pepper and old bones.

I think the trail is about a mile, but we made it only a few hundred feet before Dad was feeling tired and we had to turn around.

"Didn't we have a baby with us?" he asked as we loaded him into the car.

"Not this time, Dad," I said. "The baby's at home."

"Bigfoot!" he said, brightening. "He's not here?"

"No, he's at home with Sam," I said. "But I can bring him to see you the next time I'm here."

"Bring who?"

"The baby."

"Bigfoot?"

"Yeah."

"Never wake a sleeping baby," he said. "Just remember that."

"Okay, Dad."

We took him for ice cream at Haley's, and brought a dripping hot fudge sundae back to Al. On the drive back, Dad told me all about the people who worked at the rehab center.

"Get this," he said. "I have a male nurse. Steve. Nice guy."

"Men can do anything now," I joked, but Dad didn't get that I was being facetious, and he nodded.

"Nice guy," he said again.

Dad showed me the CD player my mom gave him, and his thick, padded book of jazz CDs. He offered me a Werther's Original caramel candy from a giant plastic bowl that was brimming with the things.

"Dad," I said, laughing, "those are old-man candies. Their commercials literally have grandpas pulling them out of their pockets on fishing trips."

"I'm an old man!" he said. "C, help me with this; I can't get the wrapper off."

My mom took a candy from Dad's outstretched, trembling hand, and unwrapped it for him.

"He just had ice cream," I said to her. "When's the last time he ate a vegetable?"

"I use these for bribes," she told me. "If he takes his medicine, he gets a treat."

"That's what you do with dogs," I said.

"Oh, Sara," she sighed, weary as hell, and I knew I'd pushed her too far. "Would you lay off? It works."

I laid off for the rest of my trip.

Over time—not enough time, really, just a few weeks—Dad lost his appetite, then lost his ability to walk on his own, even with the walker. Soon, he was too weak to do anything but yell.

We didn't understand why he was declining so quickly but thought maybe it was because being away from home made him agitated, which kept him from sleeping, which kept him from eating, which kept him from walking. We thought maybe he'd get better once he just got some sleep.

One day as my mom arrived at the rehab center, a nurse took her aside and asked her to please stop bringing the Werther's Originals, and Mom apologized profusely, assuming that maybe Dad was eating too much sugar. But the nurse said, "No, it's just that when he gets mad he throws them at us. And when he hits someone with one, he yells: 'Yeah, motherfucker!'"

"How often does he hit someone?" I asked Mom.

"More often than you'd expect," she said. "Maybe that's a good sign."

I thought so, too, but a few days later my mother called me, laughing hysterically in the same way I laughed hysterically the first time I had a Brazilian bikini wax, which was so painful that it short-circuited my brain.

"He's had a psychotic break!" she cackled. "He's a real loony tune now!"

The loony tune had woken up from a midmorning nap and thought the rehab center was under attack. He screamed, then screamed at everyone who came running that they all needed to get underground, that there were enemy soldiers outside, chipping away at the windows with knives. The center's social worker calmly helped Dad into a wheelchair and took him outside to show him that the "enemy soldiers" were actually maintenance workers, fixing some weather stripping. Dad insisted that she wheel him around the entire facility and show him where all of the doors on his floor were, so he could map out an emergency escape route.

They put Dad on antipsychotic medication.

"So that was MY day!" Mom said.

"What are we going to do?" I asked softly.

"Maybe it would be better if he came home," she said. "But I can't take him. I can't. It breaks my heart, but I can't."

"Of course you can't."

"I know everyone thinks I should take him home."

"Nobody thinks that, Mom."

"I'm doing the best I can."

"I know, Mom."

"He hates me."

"He doesn't hate you."

"It doesn't matter," she said. "It's not him anymore anyway."

The social worker told Mom that she thought my father would do better at a facility that had "memory care" services for residents with dementia. Besides the war zone hallucinations, he'd started trying to eat his TV remote control during lunch. They didn't feel that they were able to properly care for him anymore and wanted him moved. Mom agreed, and they made plans to discharge Dad ASAP so that they could give his bed to a new patient.

There were only a few such facilities that would take Medicare, so I flew home and went with Mom to check it out. This book is starting to feel like the elaborate origin story of how I reached an unprecedented level of airline elite status.

The nursing home reminded me of every movie trope that Dad's doctor, Dr. G., had told me to ignore. It was so on the nose that it *was* the nose: papery people eating soft foods with plastic spoons, some arguing about TV, some making collages with kiddie scissors and magazines, one guy yelling at an empty chessboard.

"He can't live there," I told Mom on our hugely silent drive back to the honky-tonk condo.

"Well, he can't stay in rehab," she said. "And he can't come home. He has to live there."

But that nursing home had a yearlong waiting list, and no available beds. We all braced ourselves for Dad's return home. I flew back to California.

Before he could be discharged from the rehab center, though, my poor, confused Dad ripped out another catheter tube, and it was the last straw for his immune system. He contracted MRSA, an infection that's pretty treatable if you're healthy, and excruciating, even deadly, if you're not. Instead of home, the rehab center sent him to the ER. He was hallucinating war zones again. The hospital admitted him, and told Mom that once Dad was stable they'd be bouncing him back to the rehab center. I don't understand why they took him back after they said they couldn't care for him anymore.

Dad went ballistic. He berated and threatened my mother. She refused to bring him home, and he tried to break her wrist.

"He's so angry with me," she whispered into the phone.

"What about the antipsychotics?" I asked.

"He just spits them out."

"You can't bribe him with the candy?"

"I can't do anything," she said. "He hates me."

"He's just scared," I said.

"He's dying," my mother said.

"Don't be dramatic," I said, because I didn't want to believe her. Those words were a cement block on my chest. I wasn't ready for my father to die. We were supposed to have more time. People call Alzheimer's "the long good-bye," for fuck's sake. It had been, what, a year since his diagnosis? I needed more time. He could live with me; I'd push his wheelchair and feed him the damn pudding.

"Maybe Dad will make it to his birthday," she said. "He'll be seventy this year."

"Mom. He's going to be fine."

"Remember that year you and Dan dressed up as the Statue of Liberty? Dad got such a kick out of that."

"Should I do it again this year?" I asked. "He'll think it's funny."

"We need to call your brother," she said. "You both need to come home and say good-bye."

I flew *back* to Massachusetts, this time with Sam and Colin, who was a chubby little angel person for the entire flight. I was tired of spending so much time away from him. He was rolling over now, and squealing, and making little *da da da* sounds. I've read that parents flying with small children should bring swag bags of earplugs and candy and bumps of cocaine, to hand out to surrounding passengers as a preemptive apology for loud melt-downs. Sam thought that was dumb. He told me a story about a coworker who would fly only first-class, even with his kid, and somewhere in the middle of a transatlantic flight the kid had a meltdown. The person sitting in the row behind them started to grumble about it, and then the coworker spun around and snapped: "Whatever, *sir*, if you can afford first class, you can afford noise-canceling headphones." I aspire to have the awesome confidence of a rich person who defends their children by shaming other rich people for how they do or don't spend their money.

We met my mom at the hospital, where Dad was still admitted. Mom stopped us in the hall outside his room. "He's out of his mind," she warned us. "He thinks we're under attack. Don't get too close or he might try to bite you." She handed me a few pairs of latex gloves. "We can't touch him directly, because of the infection. Make sure you put these on, and that you keep Colin away from him."

In the hospital room, Dad was agitated, confused. He looked like he hadn't showered or trimmed his beard in several weeks. He looked like he had no idea that one was supposed to shower or trim beards, or even what a "week" was. It scared me.

My Uncle Jay had flown in, too, and he was sitting quietly with Dad when we walked in. Jay stood up to hug me, shake Sam's hand, and meet his new grandnephew. Colin giggled and gurgled at this fawning new face, and Dad sat straight up like a Whac-A-Mole.

"There's a baby in here," he said.

"Hi, Dad," I said. "It's me, and Sam, and your grandson, Colin."

"There can't be a baby in here," he said. "It's too dangerous."

"It's okay, Dad," I said. "We brought Colin to see you. See, Colin? That's your Pop."

I took a small step toward my father, and my mom put a hand on my arm to warn me to take it slow.

"Say hi to Pop," I said to Colin, trying to sound bubbly. "I'm just kidding, Dad; he can't talk yet. But he's really happy to see you, and so are we. We love you so much. It's almost your birthday, you know? You're going to be seventy, old man. Let's party."

Dad beckoned me closer. I handed Colin off to Sam and moved in, holding my breath. What if my father tried to bite me? Would I get infected too? Was *this* the social disease?

Instead, he gently put a hand on my arm. "Let him live," he whispered to me, then looked down sadly at his own lap. "Let him live."

"What do you mean, Dad?" I whispered back. Did he think we were in danger? Or was this a lucid moment, and he was offering me parenting advice about allowing Colin to freely make his own decisions?

"Let him live," he repeated into his lap. Then he looked right into my eyes and said, "You're so beautiful."

"So are you, Dad," I managed.

He sighed and slumped over. I had to leave the room.

The hospital discharged my dad with an IV drip of antibiotics to try to clear out the MRSA. He was readmitted to the rehab center, into the same room, where Al was—you got it, still watching weird TV.

His first night back, Dad woke up in the middle of the night and ripped out the IV. A nurse put it back in. He ripped it back out.

"He thinks they're government tubes," Mom confided.

"What's a government tube?" I asked, like my mother would have a logical answer, like there was one anyway.

"I don't know, Sara," she said. "I don't know what he thinks is happening to him."

"Well," I said, "when he gets better we can ask him."

I'm not ready for this, I thought. *He has to get better because I'm not ready to let him go. We just need to try harder. We'll pay Male Nurse Steve to hold him down for a few days so the antibiotics work, and then when he's back to himself, Dad will laugh and say, "See? I told you he was a nice guy."*

Mom snapped me out of my delusion. "He's not getting better, honey," she said. "If there's anything you need to say to him, you should start saying it."

"What...," I sputtered, "like, now?"

"I don't know," she said, and her eyes went liquid. "Just think of every moment you have with him like it's the last one."

Chapter 19

SO THAT'S JAZZ

The military granted my brother a few days of emergency leave. He'd been back from his deployment for several months, thankfully, so he didn't need to fly in from a literal war zone—just witness Dad's war zone hallucinations.

Daniel got to Massachusetts on July 3, the day before Dad's birthday. It was weird. I hadn't seen him in a few years, and he looked like a soldier. Proud posture, close haircut, the confidence of a man who could knock you flat on your back with his pinkie finger.

We all met up in the parking lot of the rehab center, and my brother and I shared the strained embrace of mature adult siblings who will forever be irritating dum-dums to each other.

"Ready?" I asked him.

"I guess," Daniel said, and we started to head inside. Sam carried Colin a few paces behind us, so my brother and I could talk.

"Remember that movie *Happy Gilmore*?" Daniel asked. "The Adam Sandler one where his grandma goes to a nursing home and evil-mustached Ben Stiller offers her a nice warm glass of shut the hell up?"

"Totally," I said. It was one of the movies that came to mind when Dr. G. specifically told me not to rely on movies for accurate depictions of Alzheimer's.

"That's what I keep picturing," he said. "Batty old ladies sitting around making quilts, while evil Ben Stiller twirls his mustache."

"Dad has a male nurse," I said. "Steve."

"Nice guy," we said at the same time, and we laughed. We both knew our father so well.

"Do Mom and Dad mention that he's a dude every time they talk about him?" Daniel asked.

"Obviously," I said.

"Man," he said, "they're so weird. Did I tell you that Mom has started saying, 'That's jazz!' to me all the time?"

"What?" I laughed. "No. What does that even mean?"

"She'll, like, tell me that she went to exercise class and then went grocery shopping and that was her day. So that's jazz!"

"I've never heard her say that before," I said.

"She's so weird," he said. "But that's jazz!"

I waggled some exaggerated jazz hands and we laughed the forced laughs of people who are feeling each other out after a long time apart. We were still laughing when we got to our father's room and stopped short. Dad was lying on the floor wearing only a diaper, moaning in pain.

"Jeeeesus," my brother gasped.

Mom stood off to the side, chewing through her own thin cheeks, while a nurse, not Male Nurse Steve, crouched by Dad's side.

"Mom?" I asked. "What the hell's going on?"

"He fell," she whispered.

"What was he trying to do?"

Dad moaned again. He sounded like a caveman. He looked like an elderly Jesus crumpled at the foot of his own crucifix, all beard and ribs and heavy pain.

"I don't know," Mom said. "Maybe trying to get more comfortable."

"On the fucking *floor*?" I asked.

"Don't use that word," she said.

"Ira?" the nurse asked my father loudly. "Can you hear me?"

Dad tried to say something, but the words just came out garbled, like a Frankenstein groan.

Some nurses tried to delicately lift Dad from the floor. My brother started to help, but the nurse stopped him and said something about liabilities.

"He's in the *military*," I snapped. "He could lift Dad by *himself*." Mom gave me a look, and I shut my mouth.

Nobody could pick Dad up, so one of the nurses went to get a lift machine, which looked like a baby's bouncy seat hanging from the end of a small construction crane. It took a few minutes, but they got him in the seat and off the floor. Dad hung limp-limbed and helpless while they hoisted him back over to bed, and he reminded me of a cheap toy in an arcade claw machine.

Once he was settled comfortably back in bed, my mother drew a blanket over her quaking husband, and he reached up to grab her hand. We all held our breath, unsure if he would try to hurt her, but he just gave her a little squeeze and kind of danced her hand back and forth for a bit. I put some music on and Dad kept Mom's hand dancing, or maybe it was the other way around, until the movement petered out and we realized that he was asleep. Up close he looked less like Jesus off the cross and more like a caricature of a homeless man. His beard was a tangle of wild wires, his teeth thick with yellow film.

My mom saw me looking. "We've tried to use a toothbrush, Sar," she said. "He just snaps his teeth at us like a scared animal."

"Is this all happening because of the Alzheimer's?" Daniel asked. "I thought he'd just be forgetting stuff, but this seems like his body is shutting down."

"It's the MRSA," Mom said. "We can't treat it. It's so treatable, with antibiotics. But he keeps ripping out his IV, and he won't take pills, so we just have to let it run its course and hope for the best."

"He's dying," I said.

"Yes."

"I didn't believe you."

"No."

"I'm sorry, Mom."

"I know."

"What's MRSA?" my brother asked.

"It's a staph infection," our mom said, and I laughed uncomfortably loud.

"Staph," I said, "you know. Like 'staff'? Which is, like, a euphemism? For dick? Come on. We can all admit it now—Dad would think that's funny."

Crickets. Dick-ets.

He would have thought *that* was funny too.

The next day was the Fourth of July, my father's seventieth birthday. Maybe I haven't mentioned this yet? Dad's birthday was a national holiday. *The* national holiday. When we were kids Mom always made or ordered him a custom birthday cake that had nothing to do with red, white, or blue, to show him that it was *his* special day too. My favorite was a three-dimensional ice cream cake that looked like a watermelon, with layers of raspberry, lemon, and lime sorbet that she'd molded in a bowl. It had chocolate chips for seeds. Somewhere there's a photo of us the year we dressed up in homemade Statue of Liberty costumes on Dad's birthday morning, and sang "My Country, 'Tis of Thee." When Dad came down for breakfast he'd smiled widely and been totally speechless, other than a "Ha!"

This year, we'd celebrate with mini-cupcakes at the rehab center. But first, we had to make official plans for Dad's death. Death on a birthday. The timing was awful. But it was clear that Dad wasn't going to make it much longer, and Daniel didn't have any schedule flexibility.

Mom called around to a few funeral homes until she finally got someone on the phone, who told her that they were sorry, but it was both a Saturday and a federal holiday, so we should call back on Monday.

Daniel overheard our mom begging for an exception, and he gently took the phone from her. He explained, just as gently, to whoever was on the other end, that he was active duty military, that he had a limited amount of time, and that our father had even less. The funeral home immediately agreed to send someone to meet with us.

"Should we go there first?" I asked. "Or go see Dad for his birthday before we go price out his death?"

"Dude," Dan said, "that's depressing."

"It's all fucking depressing," said Mom, the first time I'd ever heard her drop an f-bomb in my entire life.

"Whoa, Mom!" I teased. "Language."

"Who fucking cares," she said.

Daniel nodded, and cracked a wide smile. "A-fucking-men."

We went to the funeral home first; a grand Georgian mansion the color of early sweet corn, with three stories of black-shuttered windows that reminded me of this perfume commercial from my childhood that made Dad laugh; it featured beautiful, furious French women in ball gowns, throwing shutters open, screaming the name of the perfume—*Égoïste!!*—then slamming them shut again. Cuckoos henpecking from their clocks.

Daniel rang the bell and the chimes must have been a hundred years old, resonating the same Gothic *BOOOOOONG-boooooong* you'd expect to hear at a haunted house on Halloween. Or, I guess, at a funeral home on the Fourth of July.

A young man answered the door, and it creaked theatrically. He introduced himself as the undertaker, but he didn't have to. His suit was comically large, his hair freshly and wetly combed close to his head. He was practically wringing his hands. I saw my brother swallow a laugh.

The undertaker welcomed us inside, and to his credit, if he was annoyed about being pulled away from a Fourth of July barbecue, he didn't show it. Instead, he led us into an ornate sitting room and gestured for us to take seats on hard, fancy couches.

When my mother was settled in, he looked at her feet and said deferentially, "Mrs. Alterman, I'm so sorry for your loss."

"Oh, he's not dead," she said. "Not yet."

"Thank you for meeting us," I jumped in. "My father's in bad shape and we wanted to all make arrangements together. My brother and I both live out of town."

"Of course," the young man said. I don't want to nickname him the "Undertaker" because there's no way I'm stepping on a professional wrestler's brand. And he was so kind—I don't want to paint him as a caricature. Let's call him Angus. I don't remember his real name, but there's no way it was actually Angus. *Are* there actual Anguses? Email me.

"That's right," Angus said, turning to my brother. "Thank you for your service, sir."

"Absolutely," Daniel said. "And thank you for helping us today."
Angus pulled out a catalog of caskets. Wow. Right to the point.

"Have you had any conversations with your husband about his wishes?" Angus asked Carolyn. "Does he wish to be embalmed? Buried? Cremated?"

"Cremated," she said, which surprised me. Not the answer, I guess, but the matter-of-factness of it. Like a diner waitress had just listed our toast options and she'd said *rye* like it was no big deal. I didn't mean to make a toast/cremation connection, it just happened organically. Sometimes the universe gives us little presents.

"Really?" I asked. "But he's Jewish."

"Not *that* Jewish," she said. "Besides, his mother was cremated too."

"But I thought Jews don't cremate," I argued.

"It's my understanding that cremation is becoming more acceptable in some Jewish communities," Angus cut in. "I've personally worked with a few families who chose cremation, and then buried the remains in a Jewish cemetery."

"Is that what he wants?" I asked my mother. "Where would you bury the remains?"

"They won't be buried," she said. "I want to scatter some and keep some with me wherever I go."

"Like...in a necklace, or something weirder?" I asked.

Angus flipped through the catalog. "We do have a lovely selection of cremation jewelry," he said. "Each piece is designed to hold a pinch of ashes. Gold...stainless steel...we may even have some rose gold options."

"Do we need a special permit to scatter ashes?" I asked him. "If we wanted to take him to, say, his favorite park, and have a ceremony outside."

"We can just do what they did in *Schindler's List*," Mom said. "I'll just put him down my pants and then shake him out of my leg while I walk. Nobody will see. That's what the Nazis did."

What?!

"*Mom*," I yelped, and Daniel looked like he wanted to die. Right place for it.

Angus, bless his face, didn't seem fazed. Maybe we weren't the weirdest, most inappropriate mourners he'd ever had to deal with. "The only circumstance I'm aware of that requires a special permit is a burial at sea," he said. "I personally haven't arranged any of those, but I'm sure someone in my family has, and we'd be happy to look into that for you."

Ultimately, we chose a simple wooden cremation casket, and a wooden urn engraved with a hummingbird. "He loved humming-birds," Mom said. "There was one that lived in the backyard of our old house, and we loved to watch it flutter while we ate our breakfast." Her eyes welled and she pinched her mouth into a wiggly line. "Sweet bird," she said. "He was a sweet bird."

"*Is*," I said. "Dad is still alive."

"He'll always be alive in my heart," she said, and Angus excused himself to go print an invoice for us. I don't remember what we talked about while he was gone, if we talked at all, but when he came back we handed him a credit card and promised to call as soon as my father was ready. Which was to say, dead.

We all stood up to shake Angus's hand, and he saved my brother for last.

"Thank you for your service, sir," he said, and slipped Daniel an envelope. "I'd like to buy you a round."

Daniel peeked into the envelope. It was brimming with cash. "Oh, thank you, but I can't take this," he said. "That's so generous of you, but—"

"Please," Angus said. "Have a drink on me. I appreciate everything you do."

"Likewise," Daniel said, and gripped Angus's hand tightly. "Happy Fourth of July."

"Well," Mom said. "Shall we celebrate?"

———

Dad's seventieth birthday was unbearable. Never mind that he was unable to move or speak or chew or swallow—the real shame was that his own family didn't bother with a special cake for what would absolutely be his last birthday on earth.

Instead, we brought supermarket mini-cupcakes in plastic cradles, frosted with stiff dollops of red, white, and blue. We barely got through singing "Happy Birthday" without all falling apart, and then Mom smeared a bit of frosting on the inside of Dad's lips so he could lick it off, and I thought about all of the cakes he'd lovingly ordered for us over the years.

The frosting smear just sat there on Dad's lips. He made some thin and throaty moaning sounds.

"Should we help him?" Daniel asked. "Dad, are you okay?"

"He's fine," Mom said. "Tastes good, huh, I? Here." She used a straw to drop some water into Dad's mouth, and the thin moans turned to gurgles.

"Oh my god!" I said. "Mom!"

"He's fine," she said again.

A nurse, not Male Nurse Steve, heard me yell, and came running. "Everything okay in here? Ira? You all right?"

"I think he's choking," I said.

"He's not choking," Mom said. "Just a little water caught in his throat."

"Drowning, then," I said.

The nurse slid an arm under Dad's neck and helped him sit up a few inches, until the gurgling stopped. She used a toothbrush to gently scrape the frosting from his mouth.

"It's your birthday, huh, Ira?" she asked loudly. "What are you today, twenty-five? Thirty?"

Dad made a single open-throated grunting sound that could have been a laugh.

"Seventy," I said.

"What?" The nurse faked it. "No way, Ira. You're not a day over thirty-five. Big plans for the day?"

"Partying hard," I said. "Want a cupcake?"

A few nurses—including *Male Nurse Steve, finally!!*, who was indeed a nice guy—gathered in the room and we handed out cupcakes and sang "Happy Birthday" again, and I tried to pretend that our guest of honor was wearing something besides an adult diaper, or at least wearing something over it.

I knelt by my dad's pillow and read him a card I'd written the night before.

My dear Dad,

Thank you. I love you. You have given me everything, and I am going to give it all to your grandson, and I am going to be ok because you helped me be ok. Thank you. I love you. I love you.

I barely got through reading that out loud, I was crying so hard. When I looked up, so was my dad.

I kissed him on the forehead, but as I was leaning in Mom whispered, "The MRSA, Sara," and I chickened out at the last second and only let my lips barely graze his skin. Then, I put the card on the rolling table, told Mom that I wanted it to be cremated with him, and I left.

I walked out on my dying father. It's the most cowardly thing I have ever done.

I understood, then, why my mom talked about Dad like he was already dead. He was gone. I'd never play dumb word games with him again, never twirl around a living room to Chuck Berry records. We'd never eat cake together, or watch innocent movies together, I'd never get another panicked computer phone call, or a sex illustration, or hear one of his bedtime stories. I'd never get to ask him about his books. I'd never get a do-over on that timid forehead kiss.

Sam, Colin, and I flew back to San Francisco the following day, and I never saw my dad again.

Chapter 20

LOVE YOU FOREVER

Ira Alterman died on July 6, 2015, two days after his 70th birthday. Ira was funny, generous, corny, and kind. He loved jazz, hiking, reading, writing, and spending time with his beloved family. He also loved terrible puns, naughty jokes, and random drives to the 24-hour L.L. Bean store. When his kids were little he'd make them play annoying word games on road trips instead of listening to music like normal people, and he always fast-forwarded through the kissing parts of movies. Ira leaves behind his wife Carolyn, son Daniel, daughter Sara, daughter-in-law Jesse, son-in-law Sam, grandchildren LaVera, Autumn, and Colin, brothers Jay and Alan, and his dog Callie, all of whom will love him forever.

Chapter 21

EVERYTHING AFTER THAT

That was my father's obituary, which I wrote ten hours after my mom called and simply said, "He's gone."

She didn't even need to say it. When I saw her name and number on my caller ID at two in the morning, I knew. I slipped out of bed, where Sam was sleeping so calmly, and tiptoed to the living room to curl up on our brown leather couch.

All I could say was, "Oh."

"It happened in his sleep," she sobbed. "A nurse went in to check on him and he was just lying there. Nobody knows when it happened. But"—and here she started sobbing harder—"he was alone."

We cried together for a minute, but then she said, "Simple."

"What?" I asked, through a mouthful of gooey sadness.

"Simple," she said again, "but elegant. Maybe a light luncheon. Finger sandwiches. Hors d'oeuvres. That kind of thing. But it has to be him. It has to be Dad."

She was talking about his funeral.

"Mom," I said darkly, "it's two o'clock in the morning, and you just told me that my father died. I will talk to you about sandwiches later."

And I hung up. It was cruel. My mom didn't have anyone else to cry to, and I had Sam.

I crawled back into bed and shook him awake.

"He's gone," I said, echoing my mother, and Sam cradled me in his arms. "My daddy," I said, choking on the word.

"Oh, babe," Sam said, and gently rocked me back and forth. It reminded me of that stupid backpacking trip so many years ago, when I got hypothermia, and he kept me safe. And I started crying harder because I thought, *Someday I'm going to lose this too.*

Sam held me until That Guy's hungry cries woke us a few hours later. We skipped work and went out for frozen margaritas as soon as any respectable frozen margarita establishment would have us, which, thankfully, turned out to be a lot earlier than you'd expect for a Monday morning.

I booked *another* flight home, for that very night. I put myself in first class, which I never did before or since, and when a flight attendant came around with cocktails, I took two from her tray, pounded them both down, and went to sleep. I awoke six hours later, bleary-eyed in Boston, and did my familiar subway/trains/sea grind that used to feel poetic and now just felt tedious.

I got off the train and automatically looked for my dad. When I remembered that he wasn't coming, that he was dead, I rolled my own suitcase along the platform, *rat-tat-tat*, and down the ramp, to where my parents' SUV idled in the parking lot. I guess it was just Mom's SUV now.

Callie tasted every crevice of my face as I slid into the passenger seat. Mom didn't seem to really notice me. She was completely glazed over by grief. I probably should have offered to drive.

I threw myself into planning Dad's memorial service so that Mom and I didn't have to talk to each other. She mostly sat staring into her lap in the living room, a trace of a sad smile on her face. I didn't know what to say to her, and I didn't really want to hear what she had to say to me. What *do* you say to someone who shares your profound grief? "Sorry for your loss"? "It's going to be okay"? Those words are all empty.

Mom didn't want a gloom-and-doom funeral that took itself too seriously, and Dad wasn't religious, so we decided to throw a party. I tried to book it at a historic inn in the 01776. There's a restaurant there that Dad loved, where the staff wears historically accurate colonial garb, and serves historically questionable iceberg wedge salads. Sometimes in high school my madrigal choir sang olde English Christmas carols in the inn's private dining room, our flushed nerd faces lit by the glow of a crackling fire.

But there was no room at that inn, so instead I found an Irish pub, located near the honky-tonk condo and a few blocks from the funeral home, that served Guinness and chowder and coconut shrimp.

I dragged Mom to a craft supply store, mostly to get out of the house, where we bought picture frames and a wooden card box with a drop slot. We planned to ask guests to write down a fond memory of Dad and leave it in the box. We went to the florist, then to Walgreens to buy a dozen bags of Werther's Originals to set out next to flowers, and photos, and a few of Dad's hats. We just occupied our days with chores we made up, to have something to do. Sam arrived with Colin, and then we occupied ourselves with the baby.

The day before the memorial I went to pick up my father from the funeral home, which sounds so casual, and on the drive over I fantasized that he'd be waiting for me on the doorstep, with two small coffees. Instead, a sweet woman met me in the foyer and handed me a plain brown paper bag that had been sitting on an antique entry table. She offered me some kind words and a warm handshake as she handed over the bag, and I was utterly confused, until I realized that Dad was in there, in a small wooden box. I wondered how much of him was in there, and if my card was in there, too, and if there were traces of anyone else's ashes that had been accidentally mixed in.

I had to make the speech at Dad's service. Mom didn't think she could speak coherently in front of a bunch of people. Daniel's not really a talker.

"I want it to be funny," I told Sam on the evening of the memorial. "Is that weird? Eulogies are so brutal. Dad would hate it if we stood around telling sad stories about him. He'd hide."

"There's this *New Yorker* article—" Sam began.

"What percentage of our conversations have begun this way?" I asked.

"—about E. B. White," Sam continued, ignoring me. "His stepson wrote it. Roger Angell. Did you know him?"

"The guy from the Who?" I asked.

"What? No."

"Are you sure?"

"Positive."

"Okay," I said. "But Roger Angell is absolutely the type of name that a guy from the Who would have."

"Anyway," Sam said, "in this article he mentions that his stepfather was a notoriously private man who hated being out in public. So when E. B. White died, Roger Angell began his eulogy with, 'If Andy could be with us today, he would not be with us today.'"

"Who's Andy?" I asked.

"That's what he called E. B. White, I guess."

"But what does the 'E.B.' stand for?"

"Elwyn Brooks."

"But then where does 'Andy' come from?"

"I don't know."

"Are you sure you have this story right?"

"Do you want me to find the *New Yorker* article?"

"No thanks," I said quickly, because that's always my answer to that question.

"My point," said Sam, "and maybe this was Roger Angell's point, is that you can make a light and funny comment about the irony of making a public speech about someone who hated public speeches, without being over the top about it."

"Am I over the top about things?" I asked.

"Only sometimes," Sam lied, kindly.

"Maybe I should just talk about *Schindler's List*," I said.

"*What? Why?*" Sam asked, and I told him about what my mom said, about the Nazis shaking ashes out of their pants.

"Did she mean *The Shawshank Redemption?*" Sam asked. "Because that's what Tim Robbins's character does with the dirt he digs out of his cell wall. Why would Nazis be shaking ashes out of their pants? There was no conspiracy to cover up the fact that they were murdering millions of people."

"So...I *shouldn't* lead off with a quote from *Schindler's List?*"

Sam shrugged. "You should say whatever you think your dad would want you to say."

At the memorial I greeted and consoled and fed Swedish meatballs and beers to about fifty people from all corners of my dad's life. Family, neighbors, work friends, college friends. His creative partner, Marty, whom I hadn't seen since I was a little girl. When I saw him, I immediately thought of the buxom cartoon on the cover of *How to Pick Up Men*.

After about an hour I noticed that people were kind of standing around uncomfortably, unclear what the mood was, wondering if they were at a ceremony of death or a celebration of life.

"I think it's time for your speech," Sam whispered to me. "I think it would make people feel more relaxed."

There's no good place to give a eulogy on the second floor of an Irish pub. I could have stood on the bar, I suppose, but it was mystery sticky and leaky tap slippery. Instead, I found a corner of the room, in front of a fireplace, and just started yelling.

"Hey everyone," I called. Someone clinked a glass, and the room got quiet. "If you don't know me," I continued, "I'm Ira's daughter, Sara. On behalf of my family we'd like to thank you for being here. Well, not all of my family. I mean, not Ira. He...didn't get to weigh in."

Nobody laughed. I took a swig from a glass of wine sitting on the mantel that was definitely not mine. "When I was trying to figure out what to say to you today," I said, "my husband reminded me of a great story from the funeral of the author E. B. White."

I told the small crowd that, just like E. B. White, my father loved his friends but hated when they gathered in groups larger than two, that underneath his groaner puns, he was actually pretty shy. I said that my dad was warm, kind, and complicated, that we had only just begun to get to know each other as people, not parent and child, when the disease got ahold of his brain. And that even after he started to decline, he was still so goddamned funny, even when he didn't mean to be. I told Mom's story about the Werther's Originals, though I skipped the "Yeah, mother-fucker," and said that we weren't there to cry; we were there to eat and drink and laugh and maybe hide out with a crossword puzzle, because that's all my father would have wanted.

We raised our glasses to Dad, and someone—I'm guessing my

brother—threw a Werther's Original at me, and it hit me directly in the boobs. It was perfect.

When it was over, back at the honky-tonk condo, my brother and I did a speed clean-out of our father's closet, stuffing endless sweater vests and pairs of pleated khaki pants into garbage bags for donation. We found Dad's wallet and three pairs of drug-store eyeglasses, we found a box of cigars and a pocket watch, we found books that we hadn't known existed, including *The Official Irish Sex Manual*, and another Bridget book.

"Oh my *god*, dude," Daniel said. "Is that *Bridget*?"

"You know about Bridget?!" I squealed.

"*Dude*," he said. "How do you think I learned about, like, *everything*?"

It was quiet in that closet for a second, and so uncomfortable. How old was my little brother when he found the books, and why hadn't he said anything?! Had Daniel processed our dad's books in the same way that I had? Did they consume and confuse him too? Did he think they were gross? Did he think they were awesome?

You know what? I didn't want to know.

"Let's never talk about this again," I said.

"Never," Daniel agreed. "Not talking. It's the Alterman way."

———

Not long after Dad died, Callie the dog died too.

One of the last walks my mom took her on was to spread some of my father's ashes along their favorite walking trail. Three ups and four downs. After that, she was acting funny, so Mom took her to the vet, where an ultrasound revealed a constellation of tumors in her belly.

Callie's death gutted my mom, who was now completely alone in the honky-tonk condo. But it brought her some peace too.

"They're together now," she told me. "They're both angels watching over us."

Mom talked about Callie's death as the first hard thing to happen after we lost Dad, and I began to track other firsts with mental notches. There were the obvious milestones, the ones I expected to hurt: the first Thanksgiving without Dad, the first Christmas, my first birthday, Colin's first birthday. But there were also small and simple firsts, and maybe those hurt the worst. Colin's first syllables, his first solid food, the first time he got scary sick and didn't even cry, just shivered and burned. I gave him droplets of baby Tylenol with a plastic syringe, and around two in the morning, when his fever finally broke, he looked straight into my eyes and laughed, then trumpeted a squishy little baby fart, and fell asleep in my arms.

Never wake a sleeping baby, I thought as I carefully transferred him to the crib. *Right, Dad?*

I remember reading somewhere that for a while after your loved ones die, you see them everywhere; their doppelgängers cutting you off in traffic or brushing past you in line for bagels. This was true for me—I felt constantly startled and confused by random bearded men wearing field hats or wool fedoras. Every time it happened I felt a swell of hope, like, maybe we were all wrong, and he was still somehow alive. Maybe this was all a joke, or a crime. Maybe his darkest secret wasn't those books, but something so sinister, he had to fake his death and hide. I'd forgive him. I miss him. It hurts.

Once, though, I really did see him, in a cozy used bookstore in Oakland. I was browsing the humor section when I spotted a first edition of *Games You Can Play with Your Pussy.*

I found you, I thought.

For the anniversary of his death, I wanted to walk a West Coast version of ups and downs. Sam and I drove to wine country so we could do some hiking and wine tasting, like civilized mourners.

We picked a random trail in Calistoga; an old mining road that climbed for nearly five miles along volcanic formations and the stone remains of a late nineteenth-century homestead. It was a scorching day, the tall trailside grass as brittle as my newly bleached-blond ponytail. I'm not usually a radical physical transformation kind of person, but it was so hard to look in the mirror every day and see my dad's nose and hair staring back at me. It's too complicated to change your nose, so I made my hairdresser take my hair as light as she dared. Crispy little wisps broke off constantly. They reminded me of what happens when you jab at dry shredded wheat with the tip of a coffee spoon.

Sam and I hiked in silence for a while. I thought I'd cry, or at least want to talk about my father the whole time. But I just wanted to get to our stopping point at a hilltop trail junction, so we could hurry back down and out of the July sun.

Why don't I feel anything? I thought. *Shouldn't this be a bigger deal? Shouldn't this feel like closure, or the end of a chapter?*

I have a close friend, Meredith, whose mother, Leslie, died two years before my dad did. They knew each other, actually, though not well. We all got together at my parents' house for what turned out to be Leslie's last Christmas Eve, and Dad's second-to-last. His penultimate. He once recommended that I start a copywriting business called "Pen Ultimate," and take on only clients who got the joke. Sorry, I'm meandering, but everything reminds me of funny little Dad things.

Dad had gotten a huge kick out of having Meredith and Leslie over for Christmas Eve dinner. "Look at all of us Jews!" he kept shouting in delight.

"Look at us!" Leslie would cry back, and then someone would yell "L'chaim!" and we'd all laugh, and then my shiksa mom brought out a huge plate of lobsters, and we went to town.

Leslie had cancer, and before she died she made it really clear to her family that she wanted to be cremated, and have her ashes spread "somewhere where things grow." Meredith and her sister figured that things grow in Paris just as well as they grow anywhere else, so a year after Leslie's death they took her to the City of Lights and had a gay ole Parisienne time. It was kind of a joke, too, because Leslie used to drive Meredith batshit bonkers by declaring things "*so Parisienne!*" with the same regularity and intensity of my dad swooning over Dunkin' Donuts.

Why couldn't Dad have left us with wishes or a plan? They didn't even have to be Paris-adjacent wishes or plans. It just would have made me feel much more connected to him. Instead, I had to wing it in the woods.

The trail spilled into swishy golden fields, and Sam and I took turns posing for pictures on a large rock overlooking the Napa Valley.

"How are you doing, babe?" he asked, swooping in for a cheek kiss and a selfie. "Do you like our nice hike?"

"I'm getting sunburned," I said. "It's hot."

"Are you feeling sad about your dad?"

"Of *course* I am," I said. "Sad, stupid, annoyed…I thought today was going to be this big event or bring a big feeling of closure. I don't feel closure. I feel sweaty."

"You sound like me, baby," Sam said, and I thought of that time early on in our relationship, when I'd begged Sam to tell me about his feelings, and he'd said he was feeling pretty hungry.

"What do you think would bring you closure?"

"Nothing," I said. "This is never going to feel closed."

———

"Boys have a penis. I have a peanut. Girls have Virginia."

This is what That Guy Colin tells me one night as I'm giving him a bath. I am wholly unprepared.

"That's kind of right," I say. "What do you know about Virginia?"

"That's where Grans is," he says, and it's true; my mother does live there, outside of Richmond. She moved there after Dad died, to be close to where Daniel was stationed with his family. "Do you have Virginia, Mama? You're a girl. Oh! No. You're not a girl. You're a lady."

It's been three years since my father died, and I'm pregnant again. This time it was happy news. This time I peed on a stick in my hometown, at Sam's childhood house. This time it was a few days before what would have been Dad's seventy-third birthday.

Colin is very concerned about how we'll get it out of my growing belly. He keeps asking: "Will the doctor have to break your tummy?" and I don't have the heart or the courage or even the first clue about how to tell him that no, actually—the baby will probably break my Virginia.

Sometimes Mom sends me boxes of Dad memorabilia as presents, stuff I've never seen before. Photos from his teenage days, his bachelor days, his early married days. Elementary school report cards and vaccination records. His first and maybe only passport. A school assignment called "A Short Short Story," written by Dad on September 10, 1958, when he was thirteen.

We moved to Perkasie five years ago, because my father got a job there. I have been going to school here ever since. My marks were not the best, but they were ok.

When I first moved here I liked baseball better than any other sport. Now I like football.

My hobby is collecting weapons. I have a German dagger and three old rifles. I also have an Indian spear.

When I grow up I want to own a chain of stores. I want to travel all around the world. I want to go to all of the famous places and see how they compare to the USA.

His teacher crossed out "to" and replaced it with "with" in red pen, and at the end of the page she'd written: "You have fewer mistakes on your paper than anyone else in the class. Next time you write on something like this, try to put down some thoughts you have about certain things."

Then there's this untitled essay from the same school year, same red-penning teacher:

I wonder what is beyond the beyond. What if we are the only human or living things in creation? If our world came to an end, what would there be? It staggers me to think what is beyond the sky. Does it go on forever, or is there another world on the other side of it? If there is nothing, what is there? If there is nothing, what will happen?

A few months ago she sent a box of letters that Dad had written to his parents from college, and they're so candid and funny, with none of the censorship that he practiced with his own kids for propriety's sake.

October 1, 1963

Dear Mom and Dad,

God! God! (and down through the major prophets of Israel, Jesus Christ, the Disciples, some Christian martyrs, and Desi Arnaz.) You don't, can't, will never, can't even hope to know what your little care package has meant to your son's ill-used stomach. My digestive juices kiss your insteps. May a thousand gift-bearing camels alight on your front lawn (although undoubtedly you would be fined quite heavily by the sanitation department.)

Nada more to report, except that I don't know what the hell is going on in math.

November 11, 1963

Dear Mom,

I went downtown tonight with the intention of buying some sort of Christmas present for my girlfriend, some sort of pin, etc. I say etc. because I actually don't know what the hell I wanted to get. I thought that some type of jewelry would be apropos. Little did I realize that I know less about jewelry than D. D. Eisenhower knows about making speeches.

So, therefore, could your eldest son make a baseless imposition upon you, which he has no right to do and if he had any respect would not even consider but which you will do anyway because you love him; but you are not sure that he knows this because you have not yet sent the food money you promised you would send and you don't think or are not sure that anyone on the verge of starvation is capable of love.

Namely, if you are going to be near a store, could you pick up
something suitable for a 17-year-old girl? I throw myself (and
my money) at your feet.

Some days I lose myself in these paper time machines. I miss
him so much; not Alzheimer's Dad, or sex-on-the-brain Dad,
but the cheddar sharp cheeseball who couldn't resist a pun. I miss
this carefree and hammy version of him, too, if you can miss
someone you never got to know.

I feel a little like I'm investigating my father by poking around
through his stuff, just like I did when I was a kid, rifling through
the bookshelves. This time there's no threat of getting caught.

The letter that stopped me slack-jawed in my tracks, though,
is typed on formal stationery, with this return address: Max
Brenner, 110 South La Brea Avenue, Los Angeles, California,
Telephone WEbster 6-7113.

Max Brenner. The fictional "candy man" Dad insisted he
worked for, whom I'd fact-checked and dismissed as a delusion.
The letter is undated, and reads:

Dear Mom et al,

Help! I am a captive in a candy house. Not physically
bound, oh no. Rather, I am held by my position, bound by my
intelligence. Allow me to explain; or perhaps you could explain
to me. Max tells me what a lucky person I am, that I am
so smart that I don't deserve to be a mere laborer. There-
fore, kindly, Mr. Brenner has made me part of management.
Doesn't that sound fine? Only, there is one small factor which
takes away from the enchantment; Max has gently broken the
news to me that management has no hours. Therefore, though I

still work for the same paltry (poultry, ie: chicken feed) wage, my hours have doubled. Tell me, Mom, is the status really worth it?

Well, how the hell is everybody back there in Perkasie, PA? I'm fine. Christ knows that i have to be.

This has been a very educational summer. For instance, just the other night, Mr. Brenner introduced me to an old and honored American institution, of which I was previously innocent. I believe Max called it "shooting craps." It was very interesting. Boy, I sure made Mr. Brenner happy He said that now he doesn't have to pay me for a month. I wonder what he meant?

What the hell, I might as well end this letter and send it already. Hello to everybody.

Love, Ira

"A captive in a candy house." When my father told this story in New Hope, and I'd fact-checked and written him off as an unreliable narrator, had that been *Dad, my* dad, breaking through the dementia? Well, even pre-dementia Dad was an unreliable narrator. But if Dad had been telling the truth about this story, and I could verify it, then maybe it would mean—

You know, I don't know what it would mean. But it would just make me feel good.

I found the contact info for Max Brenner's marketing department, and I sent them this email:

Hi there,

   This will seem like a strange email, but my late father insisted that he worked for "the candy man" Max Brenner in the early 1960s. I looked at your company history and, since your site says that the company was founded in Israel in the 1990s and that it's a made up name, I didn't believe him.

After he died we found a bunch of old letters from him to his mother, including one typewritten on Max Brenner stationery, and it's clearly very old paper and type. It mentions working for a candy company, etc. and how nice "Mr. Brenner" was. The return address was on La Brea Ave in Los Angeles.

I'm writing to you for no reason other than my own curiosity! I'm dying to know if this is just a weird and very specific coincidence, or if there's more to the Max Brenner story. I would very much appreciate any response. I'm fascinated by this family mystery.

Thanks for reading,
Sara

The very next morning:

Hello Sara!

Wow, that is a crazy story, and I completely understand the burning curiosity!

Based on what you've mentioned, I believe this is just a crazy coincidence. Anything in the 60's would be before any of our original guys started in the business, even if we only look at the ages of the founders.

The name Max Brenner is actually a combination name of the two founding partners - Max Fichtman, and Oded Brenner. I hope this helps close the mystery book!

Max Brenner International
260 5th Avenue
New York, NY 10001

I did not know how to end this book. There isn't really an end anyway. My love for my dad won't end; I don't think my grief ever will either. I'll always have unanswered questions about who he really was, and why he hid it from me, and whether I'm just being way dramatic about some campy books that aren't a big deal to anyone but me.

Toward the end of his life, Dad was obsessed with the idea of passing on a family business and leaving a legacy. I don't think it was ego. I think he was terrified that the people he loved would forget him, just like he was starting to forget us. Writing books made him feel confident and happy, and I wish I'd better supported him in that while he was still alive, instead of being distracted by my hang-ups about what I saw as my father's hypocrisy; the nerve of being a sexual person who also wanted his kids to stay kids, and to have some privacy and personal space.

As I was looking through old email conversations I had with my parents to use for this book, I found something my mom sent right after she and Dad came out to San Francisco to meet Colin. By then Dad couldn't really type anymore, but he wanted to send a story for his grandson so that someday I'd read it to him, and we could talk about his Pop. Dad knew he wouldn't be around to tell Colin stories himself.

This is my favorite of all the bedtime stories he ever told to me, "Daniel, and Fergus the Dream Gorilla," and with Mom's help, Dad rewrote it so that it stars his grandson. It's beautiful, and hilarious, and ridiculous. When I read it, I can hear my father's voice perfectly in my head. I can't think of a better legacy for him to leave.

The Boy in the Ugly Sweater

By Ira Alterman

Little Colin was really excited. It was his birthday and his grandmother had sent him a gift in a really big box.

"Oh boy!" he thought as he took off the pretty ribbons and bows and wrapping paper. "This is going to be great!"

He reached into the box and pulled out a big present wrapped in gold tissue paper. He tore through the paper and held it up...the ugliest sweater he had ever seen. "That's the ugliest sweater I have ever seen," he cried.

It had black and pink stripes going this way and that, and a big, bloodshot eye in the middle, surrounded by purple tap-dancing sheep and orange cats juggling live chickens.

To make it even worse, the next morning, Colin's mom made him wear it to school.

"It's only right," she said. "Your grandmother knitted it for you herself."

"Oh, no," thought Colin, "the kids are really going to make fun of me today."

He was right.

All he heard that day was "Hey, look at that kid's sweater," and "That's the ugliest sweater I have ever seen," and "Hey, kid, where did you get that ugly sweater?"

Even his teacher asked, "Oh, Colin, did somebody spill something on your sweater?" Teacher then realized her mistake and changed the subject.

It was the worst day of Colin's life.

When school was over, Colin couldn't get out of there

fast enough. He didn't walk home with his friends but took a back way that led him through fields and over a footbridge, and down a path by a railroad crossing. He was so miserable he almost didn't notice that a school bus filled with children was stuck on the railroad tracks at the train crossing.

"Uh, oh," he thought. "This could be a problem." It was.

At that very moment, he heard the train whistle!

The train would be coming around the bend at any moment and wouldn't have time to stop. It would plow into the bus for sure.

"Why don't you let everyone out?" he shouted at the driver.

"The door is jammed and I can't get it open," the driver shouted back.

Colin knew he had to stop the train... but HOW? He was just a little boy, and the engineer wouldn't even notice him.

Then Colin had an idea. Running as fast as he could, he flew down the tracks toward the train, taking his sweater off as he ran. He waved that ugly sweater over his head and the engineer saw it right away and hit the brakes just in time to save the bus and the driver and all the little children.

Colin was a hero.

The bus driver shook his hand.

All the children patted Colin on his back.

The engineer said, "Colin, you are a hero. You saved everyone's life, and we are all very proud of you."

"Thanks," said Colin.

"Kid," said the engineer, taking him aside. "I just have one question."

"What's that?" asked Colin.

"Where did you get that ugly sweater?"

The engineer laughed, and Colin laughed with him as he looked up at the sky and thanked his grandmother for knitting him that ugly sweater.

So, my dear Colin, remember there is beauty in everything and everyone.

Acknowledgments

Thank you to my editor, Suzanne O'Neill, who, from our very first conversation, has been incredibly generous, patient, and insightful. This book would be a completely random mess without your guidance. I'm sorry there were so many jokes about murder in the first draft.

Stacey Glick, my literary agent and friend, I'm constantly blown away by your intuition, advocacy, and encouragement. There aren't enough thank-yous for you.

Thank you for your fierce support, and fierceness in general: Meredith Goldstein, Josh Gondelman, Sydney O'Hagan, Zarrín Atkins, Casey Baker, Shirley Bartov, Emily Bergen, Laurel Bernstein, Karen Corday, Becky Girolamo, Sara Grossman, Marc Hirsh, Rebecca Jager, Neil Katcher, Suzanne LaBarre, Katie Leeman, Sally Levy Albert, Sharon McKellar, David Nadelberg, Jonathan Rand, Ken Reid, Neil Reynolds, Erika Schmidt, Sharon Steel, Shoshana Ungerleider, and Robert Woo. Jim Berry, thank you for always responding to my book-related text message inquiries within a thirty-day turnaround time, excluding holidays.

Greer Shephard, you have changed my life in the most surreal and wonderful way. Thank you for your mentorship and friendship. I'm grateful to you and Jessica Boucher every day.

Carolyn Levin, Tareth Mitch, Nidhi Pugalia, Deborah Wiseman, and Jacqueline Young, thank you for all of your hard work and support. Josh Sandler, thanks for having my back.

Thank you to everyone at The Gotham Group, especially Jeremy Bell, DJ Goldberg, and most obviously the formidable Ellen Goldsmith-Vein.

Gabrielle Birkner and Rebecca Soffer, thank you for the beautiful Modern Loss community you've created, and for the critical work you're doing to destigmatize conversations about death and grief. Dixie De La Tour, you were the first person to recognize that this weird story about my father might be interesting to other people. Thank you for your expert coaching and for putting me onstage at Bawdy Storytelling, which jump-started this whole ride.

I'm deeply grateful to Marty Riskin for being a loyal friend to my father and, now, to me. To my Uncle Jay, thank you for loving and showing up for Dad throughout his entire life.

Dan, I am so proud to be your sister.

Mom, I love you very, very, very much.

Sam, Colin, and Jacob, you are my beating heart.

Dad, joke's over. You can come out now.

About the Author

Sara Faith Alterman is a producer for Mortified, the long-running storytelling show that features adults sharing the very real, very awkward artifacts of their youth. She's written for the *New York Times*, the *Boston Globe*, *Architectural Digest*, the *Boston Phoenix*, *McSweeney's*, and Modern Loss.

Sara's a proud Massachusetts native who lives in the San Francisco Bay Area with her husband and two young sons.

A PSYCHOLOGY SERIES

Edited by

J. McV. Hunt, Ph.D.

PROFESSOR OF PSYCHOLOGY

UNIVERSITY OF ILLINOIS